A

MOTHER'S

WORST

NIGHTMARE...

READ OUR STORIES... SHARE OUR ANGELS

By:
Nicole Martin
Sharnel Williams

A Mother's Worst Nightmare...Read Our Stories, Share Our Angels©

ISBN – 13: 978-0-9898752-0-2
ISBN – 10: 0989875202

First Printing September 2013

Library of Congress Copyright Case # 1-971663841

Printed in the United States of America

Book Cover Designed by: Musa Ego Productions
Edited by: Jill Duska
Sponsored and Published by: PNG Publishing LLC

All inquiries for presentations, book signings and speaking engagements for "A Mother's Worst Nightmare... Read Our Stories, Share Our Angels" in its entirety should be sent to pngpublishing@yahoo.com.

All inquiries for individual authors can be made directly to the author, contact information is listed on each author's bio page.

A

MOTHER'S

WORST

NIGHTMARE...

READ OUR STORIES... SHARE OUR ANGELS

SHAKIL'S STORY

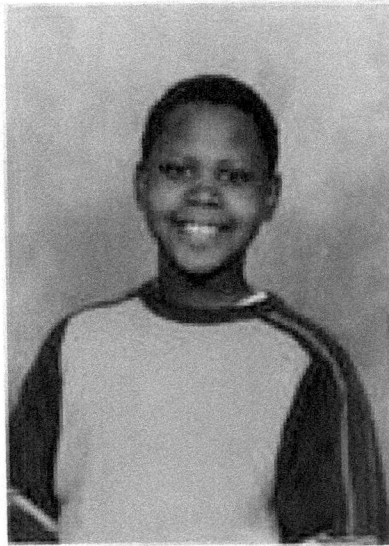

A True Story By:
Sharnel Williams

ACKNOWLEDGEMENTS

I want to thank God for giving us the strength to write this book.

Thanks to Author Nicole Martin for agreeing to work on this anthology with me.

I would like to thank my son "Kevin Williams" and husband "Kevin Brown" for being so supportive.

I want to thank my family. Without their support, I couldn't have done this.

Thanks to Mr. Joseph N. DiVincenzo (The Essex County Executive) for naming Branch Brook Park of Newark, NJ, the kids' playground, after my son.

It's called: "The Shakil Williams Playground".

Thanks to everyone who visited Shakil in the hospital.

And I would like to thank everyone who purchased this book and gave their support.

CHAPTER ONE

My son, Shakil Lennell Williams, was born in Newark, NJ on December 16, 1993. Shakil was diagnosed with leukemia in June of 2005. The first warning sign was when I noticed my son just started losing weight rapidly. I mean, within a month, he lost so much weight. He went from being husky to skinny. I followed my instinct and took him to see his doctor. Even the nurse noticed a big difference in his weight. He was only 116 pounds in March of 2005. Previously, he weighed 136 pounds in September of 2004. So as a mother, I knew something wasn't right. As his doctor looked through his chart, he kept saying he had just had a checkup in September and his blood work was normal. No! As a mother, I had to take charge and convince him to do more blood work. I told him I would feel better knowing everything was all right. Please parents, don't take no for an answer. If you really believe something is not right, pursue it.

The doctor took the blood work. He called me that

evening, and once I saw his name on the caller ID, I knew something was wrong. I was scared to answer the phone. I started getting nervous; I felt it all in my stomach.

The doctor began, *"Hello Sharnel, The blood work came back and Shakil's blood count was low; so I'm thinking that he's anemic."* He went on to say, *"He is missing his B-twelve count in his system."*

I'm thinking, *"Now, it's not that bad"*. The next words that came out of the doctor's mouth was that I needed to take my son to see a hematologist, (*a specialist that treats blood disorders*). I agreed and said I would make an appointment the next day. The doctor said that he had already made the appointment for me.

I just looked at the phone. It was Friday, and he had made it for Monday morning. I was going crazy all weekend. I felt myself getting closer and closer to my son then. I'm not saying that we weren't already close. In a time like this, you don't know what the outcome will be. I had to really show him I loved him and that I wasn't going anywhere. I was really praying that this was a dream.

CHAPTER TWO

Monday, June 6, 2005 had arrived. It was time to take Shakil to the hospital to see this blood doctor. I really was so nervous for my entire family. We walked into the doctor office, just me and Shakil. The doctor told me he needed to do some blood work on Shakil. I responded that it was fine. But after a couple of minutes, he wanted to do a bone marrow.

I was shocked! The first thing that came to my mind was cancer. My response was, *"When can I come back? Is my day off okay?"* I was off that Thursday and Friday.

The doctor responded, *"The sooner the better."*

Then I was scared! They took Shakil's blood and did a bone marrow test. Yes, all in one day! All I could do was pray. That same day before we left the hospital, the doctor set up an appointment with a gastroenterologist, (a stomach specialist).

The following Wednesday around noon, my husband and I took Shakil to the doctor. I had to leave them at the doctor's to go to work. At that time, my shift was *2 p.m.*

until 10 p.m. My son was eleven years old, and I found out he was fighting leukemia, (*a form of cancer*).

When I was told about my son, I couldn't believe it. "*Leukemia?*" I was in a daze. I can remember sitting in the doctor's office while he was talking to us, but once he said my son's diagnosis, I didn't hear anything else. As I was sitting there looking at the wall, all I could think was that maybe the doctor didn't know what he was talking about. My son was in the next room. I had to put on a strong face for him. I was the mother, so I had to be strong. The doctor was still talking, telling us what was next.

Then I heard the doctor say, "*You will have to admit him into the hospital.*"

I said, "*My son has never been admitted in the hospital before.*" This was too much going on in one day.

The doctor called for Shakil to come into the room. As he walked in, I looked at him and turned my head. I tried to hold my tears back. I couldn't; they just started rolling down my face. They were uncontrollable tears. I didn't want Shakil to see me crying, so I turned my head towards the window.

The doctor asked Shakil to sit down. I was thinking, "*This is one problem Mommy can't fix. Why?*"

The doctor was explaining to him what was going on with his health. As the doctor was talking to him, I was so nervous my stomach started hurting. When we finally left the doctor's office, crazy things started running through my head. For example:

Did something in the apartment make him sick?

Did the bowls he ate out of make him sick?

Did the water make him sick?

My mind was really racing. As we got home, I thought, "*How are we going to break the news to my oldest son?*"

The doctor let us take him home for the weekend. He was going to admit Shakil the following Tuesday. Knowing we had to take him the following week to stay all night in the hospital, my heart was in so much pain. I couldn't believe my family was going through this. I wouldn't wish this on my worst enemy.

We tried to live as we normally did that weekend. It was so hard for me. *How can a mother live normally after the news she had just received about her baby?* I think I was more nervous than any family member. Crazy things were running through my mind all weekend. I asked myself, "*Why is this happening to us? Did I do something wrong and karma is coming back to bite me? Wow!*"

Finally it was Tuesday. As we entered the hospital and sat down in the admitting area to wait on his room, I started talking to Shakil about why he was there. I reassured him that everything was going to be okay. I was so nervous! For one thing, Shakil never had to be admitted in the hospital for anything. This was something new for him and also for the family. I was the only one out of our family who ever stayed in the hospital, and that was only because I was having a baby. Everyone kept telling me, "*If you pray, everything will be okay.*"

CHAPTER THREE

Let me tell you a little about my son. Shakil won the Fishing Derby of Essex County eleven times. He was a normal child. He loved watching wrestling, playing football with his friends, and he really loved video games. He loved the video games so much that he would cry when he lost. I can envision myself saying, *"Boy, it's just a game!"* If you had a chance to get to know him, you would have loved him too.

They let us know his room was ready, and as I got up to the floor, it hit me. Wow! As I walked down the hall, there were a lot of sick kids younger than my son. I started feeling selfish, because I wasn't the only parent that had a sick child lying in the hospital. As we went into the room, I started looking around. I asked myself if I did the right thing by taking him to see his doctor. If so, why did I feel so bad? Damn!

The next day, they wanted to start everything. He had to go to the operating room; they wanted to do a spinal tap and put in a catheter. A couple of days after that, they wanted to start chemotherapy. Before the doctor started with chemo, he sat us down and told us about the side effects. He warned us about the vomiting, loss of appetite, and the fact that Shakil would most likely need a lot of blood transfusions. I just started thinking, *"What are they doing to my baby?"*

Everything the doctor said was true. One week later, Shakil lost his appetite, and the following week, he started losing his hair. I was wondering if the doctor got his paperwork or blood work mixed up with someone else's. Seeing my son sick, I was so unhappy. He wasn't eating and his hair had started falling out. As a mother, I couldn't do anything, and I felt so helpless.

A couple of weeks later, Shakil started running a fever. We found out he had an infection around the tube, meaning the catheter. The doctor had to put him on antibiotics and stop his chemo for a week. A couple of days later, they took him off one of the antibiotics. I learned they had him on three different ones to see which one would work faster.

My son was aware of everything that was going on. As parents, I think we should tell our child the truth about his illness. We were really honest with him, which played a big role in trust. If your child can't trust their parents, who can they trust?

They finally took him off of all the antibiotics, since his fever was gone. One thing I learned from my son losing his appetite is that if someone loses their appetite; don't try to make them eat because they will just get upset. And they don't need to be stressed. They have a lot going on. As a parent, we should try and make the child more relaxed and comfortable. I was so worried about him not eating, and it was getting to me, not realizing that the loss of his appetite came because of his illness. I didn't want him to get sicker by not eating anything. You know if you don't eat all day, it makes some people catch a headache or feel weak.

But the doctor said it was okay that he didn't eat at that time. I had to make his room feel like home and his bedroom. We brought his games and DVD player to the hospital. He really enjoyed having his things there. He would play his game every day, as long as he felt up to it. He met two friends in the hospital. They used to come to the room and play cards and the video games with him. Both of them had leukemia too. One had the same as my son and the other had a different kind of leukemia.

We started talking to the parents and getting to know one another. Sorry to say, both of those kids are no longer with us. I wish I could reach out to their parents today. God bless them!

It was a bad time for my son to be in the hospital. For one thing, it was summer time. I feel as though no child should have to spend their summer months in a hospital bed. A child should be out enjoying the summer with their friends and family. I felt so bad for Shakil, but I just couldn't do anything.

It was July 4th. Every year we would go to Liberty Park in Jersey City, NJ to see the fireworks. But not this year. My son was lying in a hospital bed fighting for his life. We couldn't even see the fireworks out the window.

We heard it, but the view was bad.

The next day, I was feeling bad. I know Shakil felt bad too. I wanted to ask him about the previous day, but I didn't. He would always lift my spirits when I saw that smile on his face, and until this day, when I look at his picture and I'm having a bad day, his smile will make me smile. I really believe if it wasn't for my son being sick, I would not have prayed liked I prayed. Because of my son, I believed there was a God. I believed it before, but not like when he was fighting cancer. I prayed and started looking at church on TV. I mean, I really started getting into church TV.

Shakil had lots of visitors in the hospital. He was happy when someone came to see him. Even the Mayor of Newark, Cory Booker, came to see him. He played cards and talked to my son a couple of times. He was running for Mayor at the time. He might not even remember, but we do.

One day I asked the doctor if Shakil could come home for the weekend. I was surprised when he said yes. He had been out twice already on weekends. I saw a smile on Shakil's face when I told him. I can still see his smile, brightening up the whole room. For me, as long as my baby was smiling, that made my day.

Shakil started getting another fever and losing his appetite again. They had to give him some Tylenol once again, and then his fever started coming down. With this illness, I was learning something new every day. A week later, they did another bone marrow on him. There was good news: the chemo was working. I shouted out,

"YAY!" When the doctor told me, I knew there was hope. I continued praying. I just knew that God was hearing me. I was so happy, I wanted to celebrate.

The doctors wanted to continue with his chemo, but his blood count was too low; they had to wait until it came back up. Damn! While waiting for his blood counts to come back up, Shakil caught another infection. Those damn infections was getting on my nerves!

The infection, took place again around his tube. I started thinking that as soon as things started going well, then something else went wrong. Cancer is a very powerful disease; it knows no color. Because of the infection, the doctors were talking about removing his tube once again. They were thinking about putting the tube in his arm until his chest healed. Once his chest healed, they would take it back out and replace it back in his chest. That was too much sticking to me. The problem I had with this situation is that they had to keep putting him to sleep to do this.

The next day they took him back to the emergency room. They brought him back to the room thirty minutes later. They were unable to find a vein, so they would have to try again the next day. *See what I mean?* All this getting put to sleep was starting to bother me. Once a nurse entered the room, I talked to her about the danger of getting put to sleep back to back. Her response was that they had to do it so he could get better.

I truly felt that the doctors were making my baby sicker. In my opinion, Shakil was okay until I brought him for another checkup. I just had to see why he was losing so much weight. The diagnosis was leukemia. I was stressed out at this point.

I had a routine, back in forth to the hospital. My work hours were from 2 p.m. - 10 p.m. I would leave my job and go straight to the hospital. On my days off, I would stay at the hospital and my husband would go home and get some rest. He would be in the hospital all week with Shakil. He took a leave of absence from his job. Trust me, this was not easy, but someone had to continue paying the bills. We didn't want to be homeless on top of everything else.

Weeks went by, Shakil started eating again and playing around. That was the Shakil I knew before he became ill. They took him back to the emergency room to try and put the catheter in his hand. That was successful, no problem.

CHAPTER FOUR

Two weeks later, my baby went back to the emergency room to put the catheter back in his chest. They decided to do everything at once this time. The doctor wanted to do a spinal tap and a bone marrow too. Everything turned out fine. The next day they started the eight day chemo. I was there to see them start him on the chemo, but I had to leave and go to work.

That night after work, I couldn't wait to get back to the hospital. Once I opened the door, his smile made me smile. I left around 1a.m. to go home. An hour later, my husband called me and said that Shakil had a fever. I couldn't believe it! He was just playing around and laughing with me. I asked him how high the fever was.

He said, *"High."*

"How high?" I persisted.

"One hundred and four," he replied.

Cancer…the things your body goes through trying to fight this disease! Thank God his fever did go down! My husband called and told me the news. The next day Shakil started feeling weak. He hadn't eaten or drank anything in the last couple of days.

When the doctors came in to check him, they decided it was time to feed him through an IV. Damn! Things really started getting crazy. Later on that night, the doctor had told us that Shakil was losing potassium.

I asked, *"Why is he losing it, what's going on?"*

The doctor explained to us that not having enough potassium could affect his kidney. I kept blaming the doctors for everything. Yes, I was playing the blaming game, but it actually wasn't a game. This was real life. Now when the blood transfusion kicked in, he needed two pints. I kept praying, hoping I would wake up and find out that it was all a dream.

The following week, the doctors needed to talk to us. All I could think of was what would come next. They told us to come out in the hallway; they didn't want to talk in front of Shakil. They said that Shakil was going to need a bone marrow transplant.

At that point, I was tired of asking questions. It seemed like every week, they were telling us something new. They tested the immediate family: me, my husband, and my other son. None of us were a match, I thought that was odd. We had to go to a different hospital where they specialized in that kind of surgery. I made the appointment for the following week. I was so frustrated; I didn't want to see another doctor. The day of the appointment, I was so tired. I kept asking God to lead us in the right direction. I mean, I prayed on this, I really prayed.

As Shakil slept, I sat by his bedside and just stared at him, asking God if I did something wrong. *"Why is my baby battling leukemia?"* I would also talk to God and ask Him, *"Will he be okay?"* No matter how my son felt, I would always ask him, *"How do you feel?"*

No matter what he was going through, he would say, *"I'm good."*

As a mother, I was hoping that I could have done something. But it was all in God's hands. I felt so helpless and stressed out because it was out of my hands. Mothers are supposed to be there for their kids, nurture them when they are sick, give them a hug when they need it. I was thinking about what type of mom I was. I was a great mom; I was there by his bedside. He knew I loved him and still do. Please don't take your kids for granted. It hurts me to my heart when I hear that a parent killed their child/children.

On day eight of his chemo, he again started getting a fever and he was still not eating on his own. They took him off the liquid food, but he still wasn't eating. Then he needed platelets.

I asked, *"What the hell are platelets?"* I never heard of it before.

The nurse brought the bag in the room and showed me. It was a clear bag with yellow fluid in it. They had to give him two pints.

My son was up there fighting for his life. I realized that the following week was his fishing tournament. We were hoping that he would be able to go.

We had to go to a different hospital to talk to a doctor

about the bone marrow transplant. Once we got there, we met with the doctor that was in charge. He just explained about finding a donor and adding his name to the donor list. He talked about the surgery and about how long he will be in the hospital. That was only if everything went all right. At that time, I still believed that everything would be okay.

A lady came to see my son. She said that she heard about his illness through a friend of hers. She said that she would pray for him. I was told that not everybody's prayers were good for you. I thanked her anyway for taking the time out to come see him. Before she left, she told me to continue praying.

As she was walking out the door, she said, *"Everything happens for a reason."* I looked and started wondering, *"Who is that lady?"*

CHAPTER FIVE

Shakil started eating a little, and his fever went away, but then he was vomiting and feeling bad. I asked myself, *"What's next?"* It just seemed like things weren't getting better.

Day eight of his chemo was finally finished. We were waiting on a donor. He missed his fishing tournament; he wasn't feeling good that day.

Everything started going in our favor. He was up playing his game every day and he had a little appetite. The thing I loved is that he started smiling again. You probably wonder why smiling means so much to me. I can't explain it, it's just that when he smiled, I felt this warmth come over me. Until this day, smiling is so important to me - no matter what (smile)!

Since Shakil was feeling better, I asked the doctor if he could go out on a day pass. He checked Shakil out and said, *"Why not?"*

All of us had smiles on our faces. He was so happy to see the outside; all I can do was look at his facial expression. That was a Kodak moment. We only had two hours outdoors. We went to his favor place, the park. He wasn't up to being in the park though, so we left. We headed home, and as we were parking the car, his friends ran up to the car. Yes!

Shakil had a big Kool-Aid smile on his face. A couple of hours went by, and then it was time to take him back to the hospital. We were all sad at this time and we just wanted all the drama to go away.

Two days later, Shakil started losing his appetite again. He was at the point where he started hating the smell of food.

One day I brought my sandwich in the room. He said, "*Mom, can you take the sandwich out of here?*" It was making him sick to his stomach.

I used to feel like that when I was pregnant with him. I couldn't stand the smell of chicken. It made me feel like I was going to vomit. So I ate my food in the hallway. I asked the doctor about Shakil getting sick from the smell of food and he said it was normal.

Shakil finally started feeling better again, and he was up and laughing. The following weekend was the big Labor Day festival, when a lot of people go to the park and have fun. The big parade would be that following Sunday. I was waiting to talk to the doctor about going to the festival for the weekend. He finally came to the room and I asked him. He said he didn't see a problem.

Friday afternoon, Shakil was discharged for the whole weekend. I was excited to have him with me. We went to the mall to do a little bit of shopping. We went to a couple of stores, and then Shakil started feeling tired. That was not my Shakil. He would have been excited to be in the mall. He loved going to the mall because he would always get something. That day, we had to sit down on the bench twice. I finally told him we were leaving.

That was one of my wake-up calls, the fact that my baby kept getting tired. He just didn't have the energy to walk the mall. The next day, we got up to get ready to go over to the park. Luckily for us, the park was right across the street from our apartment. As soon as we arrived in the park, everyone started shouting for Shakil to go out on stage.

We sat down, and Shakil leaned over and asked me, *"Why everyone keep looking at me?"*

"They know you are sick. And some people that know you can't believe it."

Walking toward us was his best friend and his mother. They lived in our building. Shakil was so happy to see them, I think because he had someone to talk to. I was happy too; they been at the hospital since day one. It was good to have someone to talk to in a situation like that. Shakil's friend's mother and I became the best of friends, and until this day, we still keep in touch. We had a nice time at the park. The next day we went to the parade, and Shakil was smiling from ear to ear.

The following week, we had to take him back to the doctor so the doctor could check his blood count. His count was okay, so they let him stay home a couple more days. I was happy; I had my smile on my face! At the time, we were living in New Jersey but planning on moving to Pennsylvania. We received a phone call from the builders. They said we needed to come to PA to pick out the colors and other things we had to do for the house.

The call came on time. Shakil was home, so I planned to take the trip up there the next day. I called it our road trip for the day. As we were riding up, we were taking pictures of the mountain, which was a pretty sight to see. As we pulled up to the building, we were all excited. We were actually buying a house!

We entered the building and waited for the lady to bring us into the office. She started showing us the cabinets. Shakil picked out everything, from the inside to the outside. My husband and I just sat back and let him do his thing, and in doing his thing, he did a nice job.

I remember a moment as we were driving back to Jersey. Shakil asked us, *"Can I have a lock on my door?"*

I turned around and looked at him in the back seat. I said, *"Denze..."* It was our nickname for him, short for Denzel. I wanted to name him Denzel, but my husband said, *"You are not naming him that!"* My oldest son came up with the name Shakil, but I still called him Denze from time to time. So my eleven-year-old son asked for a lock for his bedroom door. I asked him, *"What you need a lock for?"*

He responded that my oldest son kept touching his belongings. I started laughing, but he said, *"I'm for real, Mom!"*

I will never forget that moment. We had always lived in a two bedroom apartment. They always had to share everything in the room. I was glad they were finally getting their own rooms.

Returning home, we pulled up to park our truck. Shakil's friend ran up to the car. They asked his father if he could go outside. His father asked Shakil if he was tired, and Shakil said he was not. I asked him if he wanted to stay outside, and of course he said yes. As a mother, I wanted to make him happy. He'd been in the hospital all these months; I knew he needed some friend time. But I was thinking that it was a long day and he needed to get some rest. I really didn't agree with him staying outside. Shakil still had the catheter in his chest, which was another reason I didn't want him outside. At the time, I was just being a concerned mom. He stayed outside, and I was so nervous! For one, he loved playing football. I was thinking about what would happen if the ball hit him in his chest. Things were running through my mind. I kept looking out the window at him playing.

At one point, I thought I heard him calling me. I looked out the window and didn't see him. I started calling him, and he answered, *"I'm playing in the hallway!"*

I yelled out, *"Are you okay?"*

He said, *"Yeah, Mom."* He said it like I was bugging him. I was a concerned mom; do you blame me?

CHAPTER SIX

It was time to take him back to the hospital. Time sure does fly when you are enjoying your life. Two weeks later we held our first blood drive. That was the biggest turnout they ever had in Newark, NJ in one community. I want to thank everyone for their support.

One week later, it was time for chemo again. I was thinking, *I hope I don't have to go through Shakil not feeling well all over again.* I could hope, anyway!

After a couple of days, Shakil started to get nauseous. It was hard watching my baby go through this illness. If God would have told me, *"Everything will be all right, I will make Shakil better, but you will have to pick up where he left off. Meaning that you will have leukemia."* Without hesitation, I would have said, *"heal my son."*

Shakil was vomiting and not eating. One week later, his blood count went down. He needed a blood transfusion and platelets. He was having loose bowel movements. He kept screaming, *"My stomach hurts! My stomach hurts!"*

I had to call a nurse into the room and tell her what was going on. She went to call the doctor. He entered the room about fifteen minutes later. He examined Shakil, and his diagnosis was that he had cramps.

You should have seen the way I looked at the doctor. I said, *"Cramps?"*

He simply said, *"Yes."*

His pain was so severe; all I heard was Shakil yelling! Watching my son screaming like that was upsetting me because I couldn't take his pain away. The doctor gave him something for the pain and it put him right to sleep. As a mother, I was glad he went to sleep. You don't want your child sick or in pain.

The next day, Shakil started running a fever again and losing his appetite. I was getting to the point of asking myself if he was getting better or worse. It seemed like one week he was okay and the next week he was feeling bad. It was a win/lose situation. So he didn't have any appetite, he was running a fever and vomiting. He had diarrhea too.

The doctor decided to give him some medicine called morphine. I asked the doctor if Shakil was too young to get that type of medicine.

He said, *"Don't worry, it will be a low dosage and it will make him relax and feel much better."*

I was skeptical because I had heard crazy things about morphine when an adult took it. The doctor also gave him some medicine to stop his diarrhea. I just prayed and asked God to watch over my son. He still had no desire to eat, but the medicine the doctor gave him for the diarrhea was working, at least. The next day, Shakil needed two bags of platelets. He slept the whole day off and on. The morphine was working, I guess. The morphine started giving him a side effect. My son was looking at the window and he said he saw clowns on the window. Yes, he started hallucinating! I had to call the nurse in the room; I didn't know what was going on. All I knew was that I didn't see any clowns on the window. The nurse came in and said she'd have to call the doctor. The doctor finally came to his room. At that time, Shakil was asleep again. He started telling us what was going on. He confirmed that Shakil was hallucinating. I asked why, and he blamed it on the morphine. The doctor said he would take him off. I was so scared; I thought he was going crazy. I was thinking all that medicine they gave him had started messing with his brain. Once Shakil woke up, he was all right.

The next day as I was washing Shakil up, I noticed a bump by his rectum. I asked the doctor about it, but he said it was nothing and that it would go away, there was nothing to worry about. He never told me, what it was.

Shakil was up, feeling much better, and I was too. If you don't know, there are a lot of ups and downs which come with fighting cancer. It was the smile; my baby was smiling again. That smile really made my day.

Shakil's counts were still down. They decided to give him a shot in his leg with some type of medicine. The medicine was supposed to help his blood count come back up. I was hoping that the medicine worked. His blood count had been down now for a couple of weeks now. I was just praying on it.

I asked the doctor if Shakil could come home for the weekend. I knew he needed to get out and get some air. The doctor wanted to see if the medicine would start working first.

A couple of days later, he came into the room smiling. He said, *"Yes he can go home for a couple of days."*

We were happy, and we started planning things to do.

That Friday, at 10:00 a.m., the doctor gave us the discharge paper. At 11:00 a.m., his mouth started bleeding. He had sores on his lip already. I thought it was coming from there. There was so much blood. I ran out of the room to get the nurse.

The nurse came in and said, "I will call the doctor." She handed me some towels and said, *"Put it by his mouth."*

I'm telling you, there was a lot of blood! The doctor showed up and said, *"What's going on, Shakil?"* He examined him and said - now get this - all of the blood came from a loose tooth.

I looked at the doctor again; I call it my crazy face. I said, *"Are you sure all this blood came from a loose tooth?* He said yes, and then he said Shakil might not be able to go home. I wasn't really upset about that; my son's health came first. He had to give Shakil two bags of platelets and keep an eye on him.

The bleeding finally stopped but the doctor still didn't want to take a chance sending him home. I still couldn't believe all that blood came from a loose tooth. I had no choice to go by what the doctor said. It had been a couple of hours, and Shakil said he was feeling good.

It was around 9:00 p.m. when the doctor came to check on Shakil. He said everything looked good. The next thing that came out of his mouth was, *"Shakil, you can go home."*

I looked at him and said, *"Now?"*

The doctor said yes. We were happy all over again. I got him dressed and we were out of there.

Shakil's appetite still wasn't good, but he was eating a little. The next morning I wanted to take him to see family members, so we went to a couple of their houses. He enjoyed himself. The following day his father took him and his friend fishing. He had the whole weekend to do whatever he wanted to do. After they came back from fishing, he took a shower and wanted to eat. I asked him what he wanted to eat. If you remember, he wasn't eating that much. So, when he said he wanted to eat, I felt good about that. I asked, *"What do you have a taste for?"*

He said, *"A hot dog."*

I looked at him in surprise. *"A hot dog?"*

He said, *"Yeah."*

Well, I took the hot dogs out and put them in a pot. I was happy that he was a little hungry. He could have eaten anything that night; I was just thankful.

CHAPTER SEVEN

Monday, he had to go get a check-up. They wanted to see if his counts were coming back up. The doctor said his count came back up just enough to start chemo. He wanted us to bring him back to the hospital the next day. Oh boy!

We went back to the hospital. The doctor came in the room and was happy to see Shakil. He was asking him what he did at home. Shakil was talking to him and laughing. The doctor decided to do the chemo the following day.

School had started back up. There was no way he was going to school. Shakil had to get a tutor twice a week. It worked out for a couple of weeks, and then he started feeling sick again. We had to stop the tutoring for a while, right when Shakil was just getting to know the tutor. Once again he lost his appetite and started feeling weak.

I started talking to God and asking. *"Why is this happening to my son?"*

My son was a good child, never disrespected anyone. I never had to come to school and talk to his teacher about his behavior. I mean, I'm not saying this just 'cause he's my child. Anyone who got to know him knew he was a good child.

On the last day of his chemo, he started feeling nauseous. It would usually take him like a week to get sick. The following week, they had to put him in ICU. The doctor explained to me why Shakil had to go there. The chemo he just completed was a special type of chemo, so they needed to watch his heart rate. I asked the doctor why he didn't tell me that before he did this "*special type of chemo*". I just couldn't wait until this was all over, meaning my baby was cured and he could go home. Shakil's counts started going back down. He was up playing his game all that day. He had all the games that came out. My son was spoiled!

It was Halloween and Shakil was still in the hospital. The nurse told him he could walk around on the floor. The nurses were passing out Halloween candy. It still wasn't the same as walking the streets and knocking on people's doors. He enjoyed himself anyway. I think I was sadder for him than he was. We just had to take it one day at a time.

Shakil was in ICU for a couple of weeks, but finally it was time for him to go back to his regular room. It was much better, because in ICU, he was only allowed two visitors at a time. In the regular room, it was more like six people at one time. He was back to feeling better again. He had visitors every day. He was glad to see everyone.

One week later, he started having a little fever. They had to do an X-ray on him, so they took him to the X-ray room. It was always something. This disease will have you going crazy. It takes a lot of patience to deal with this. As a mother, I was stressed out.

I was at home when my son called me. I said to him, *"What's up, Shakil?"*

He said, *"Mom, my nose is bleeding!"*

I asked, *"Where is your father?"*

"He went downstairs to the store."

It really surprised me that he left Shakil by himself. He would always say he didn't want him alone. I told Shakil I was on my way. As I was driving, I was thinking it was nothing. I thought it was just a normal nosebleed.

But when I entered the room, there was blood everywhere. It was all over the sheets. That wasn't a normal nosebleed; there was too much blood for that. The nurse was cleaning him up. Around one hour later, Shakil started vomiting blood. There was so much blood coming up, you wouldn't believe it. Blood clots started coming out of his mouth, lots of them. I was so afraid he was going to go into a shock. He lost a lot of blood - I mean a lot.

His father walked into to room and asked what happened. We were waiting to see the doctor so we could get to the bottom of it. I was afraid. The nurse had saved some of the blood in a bed pan. She wanted the doctor to examine the blood.

Finally, the doctor was there and he was ready to look at Shakil. By that time, he had stopped vomiting. The doctor completed his exam. He said his diagnosis was that it was just a nosebleed. Now, y'all know my look. I looked at him like he was crazy again.

I said, "A nosebleed? There was too much blood for a nosebleed. Anyway, the blood was coming from his mouth, not his nose." And to make it worse, it wasn't even Shakil's regular doctor. It was an intern. I shouted out, *"I need a real doctor! Can someone call my son's doctor? I need to speak to him now!"*

I was so upset! I couldn't believe I was talking to an intern. There's nothing wrong with an intern, but I wanted my son's doctor; he knew what was going on.

He was there since my son was first admitted. No, I didn't want to speak to another doctor, intern or not. I wanted to talk to my son's doctor.

The intern wanted to explain why this happened. He said it was a nosebleed and the reason he was vomiting was because he was holding his head back. The blood was dripping down into his stomach. The blood didn't have any place to go but sit there. That's why he started vomiting; it had to come out. It started making a little sense.

CHAPTER EIGHT

A couple of hours later, Shakil started vomiting again. This time his doctor was there to see it all. The doctor said he had to call the Ear, Nose and Throat doctor. About thirty minutes later, the specialist came in. Shakil was examined by the doctor. The doctor stuffed his nose with cotton and gave him some kind of medicine for his nose. A couple of days later, Shakil was feeling much better. They wanted him to go and take an X-ray the following day. The result was in: he had an infection in his lungs.

He had a couple of infections since he'd been in the hospital, so to me, it wasn't any biggie. That was one thing about fighting this disease which the doctor warned us about: the infections. He needed a blood transfusion and platelets.

Every mother has a goal in life for their child to succeed in life. Well, my goal was for my son to beat this thing called cancer/leukemia. They would always give him antibiotics. We had just found out the girl that used to play cards with my son had passed away. The nurse told us. I didn't know how to tell my son. Once we came back from viewing her body, we told him. That was so sad.

A couple of hours later, Shakil started vomiting. I kept thinking about the girl. The doctor had to rush Shakil to ICU. The same situation happened to the girl; she was vomiting blood and they had to rush her to the ICU too.

They had to monitor Shakil's heart rate and blood pressure. Remember, a couple of weeks ago they said his heart rate was low. He started running a fever, so the nurse gave him some Tylenol. His fever started coming down, but he was still feeling nausea.

The doctor ordered an EKG and another X-ray for the following day. After the results came back, it showed his heart was a little abnormal. Damn! It was always something. The doctor said he was going to start him on some heart and blood pressure medicine.

I sat by Shakil's bedside and asked him, "*How do you really feel?*"

His response? "*I'm good.*"

No matter what, he was a fighter, I mean a real trooper. All I was thinking was that they were killing my baby slowly. All this medicine they were giving him was messing with his heart, and that wasn't good. Shakil had started coughing a little at first. As the weeks went by, he started coughing more than usual. The doctor checked out his coughing. Days later, they took him for another X-ray and a CAT scan. All I could do was pray and ask God to look over him.

It was time to see what type of infection Shakil had. I didn't know there were so many types of infection. I was learning different things every day. The doctors explained that the only way to find out what type was to cut him open. Now they were getting ridiculous. They were talking about cutting now. I was really starting to think I needed to get a second opinion.

My husband called a doctor at St. Jude's Children Research Hospital. He spoke to someone in that line of work. He had to update him on Shakil's situation. He told my husband that the only way to find out what type of infection they were dealing with was to cut him open and do a biopsy. So my husband and I had to really sit down and talk about it.

The next day, all different types of doctors wanted to talk to us, heart and lungs specialist plus others. There were like ten of them around the table. I knew this was serious, but I had questions, and I wasn't leaving that table until I got answers. They poisoned my son's body with all that medicine. Now he was having so many complications. It was my duty as a mother to get all the facts.

They were telling us that the surgery would be complicated, so we had to prepare ourselves for the worst. They let us know that once he got out of surgery, he might have a breathing tube in him. The main thing that stuck in my head was that he might not make it out of surgery. They really laid it out on the table. Wow! They really gave us something to think about.

The next day, we agreed to the surgery. I was so

scared; I was up all night. But thankfully, the surgery was a success. Shakil had no breathing tube, and his eyes were opened. He just had a small cut by his side. We were even talking to him. The doctors were really surprised about the outcome. I think they were looking for the worst.

The blood counts were low, and we needed them to come back up to help fight the infection. They had put him on some medicine, hoping it would help. All we could do was pray; that was our last hope.

The doctor informed us that his counts continued to be low. The doctor told us about a new treatment which was out. It wasn't approved yet by the FDA. I wanted to know a little more about the new treatment, so my husband called the doctor back at St. Jude's. We wanted to get some information about it.

The doctor from St. Jude's explained that it would help the counts come back up and kill the cancer cells, something like that. But the only thing was that since it wasn't approved by the FDA, if we decided to try it, it would be at our own risk. That was something else to think about. Being in that hospital, all I was doing was thinking. I was thinking about this, thinking about that.

As a mother, I just wanted my son to get better. We didn't do the treatment, so I would never know if it would have worked.

A couple days later, they wanted to do another X-ray to see if the medicine was helping. They did the X-ray, and everything was still the same. Damn! The doctor said that if his counts came back up, he had a chance to fight this, but he couldn't fight it while his counts were so low.

I started praying again; I was praying every day and night. I was praying before this happened, but not every day. To tell the truth, I would only pray when something happened. I know; you don't have to say a word. I learned my lesson. Now, praying is a must for me. Don't wait until something happens to get your pray on. Pray!

CHAPTER NINE

Shakil put up a good fight; he fought with us by his bedside. His oxygen level went down a little. The doctor told us that he must get air into his lungs and that the only way to do that was to get him an oxygen mask. It was looking bad, in my eyes. All I could think about was that his oxygen level was dropping. He was still in ICU. Once they put that mask on his face, he looked so sick. My baby wasn't getting any better. Do you know it hurts so bad to see your child sick when you can't do anything to make it better? He was hurting physically and mentally, and I was hurting mentally also.

There was a doctor who worked in ICU who asked us to come in the hallway to talk. He asked us how we were holding up, and then he said we needed to prepare ourselves. He told us something no parents want to hear. He told us about the type of infection my son had and said no child had ever survived it.

I said, *"There's a first time for everything. What, am I supposed to stop praying?"*

He said, "*No, keep praying.*"

I looked at him like he was crazy. The doctor was still going on about the kind of infection my son had. He said his counts were too low to fight off this type of infection. I said to the doctor, "*You are not God.*"

I just went back into the room with my son. Time was being wasted talking to that doctor. I did think about what he said as I looked out the window. I said to my husband, "*How does man tell you to prepare yourself? Man is not God. When God gives me a sign, I will.*"

My husband told me I was in denial. We talked about what the doctor said. My husband said, "*He has been a doctor for years; he knows what he is talking about.*"

That went in one ear and out the other. He said I needed to face reality; my son was not going to survive this. I was mad at him as a husband and a father. I said to myself that a doctor can tell him anything. I went into the hallway and started crying. I realized my son was still breathing, so why was I in the hallway crying? There is a word called miracle. I felt by me crying I had declared him dead already.

Shakil started getting weak; he started using a bed pan. I still prayed. I believed you have to go through the pain to get better. Maybe I was in denial, but I wasn't settling for what the doctor was saying. Everyone knows this quote: "*It is what it is.*" I hated when my husband used to say that to me. Until this day I, don't use that quote; I hate it. I know hate is a strong word, but that quote will never come out of my mouth.

Around November, Shakil started getting more blood

transfusions and platelets than usual. He really started getting sicker. I was crying so much. I started thinking to myself, *"What are they doing to my baby?"* To me it seemed like before I brought him to the doctor, he was all right. Yes, he was losing weight, but he wasn't sick in my eyes. He was going to school like a normal child does, playing outside with his friends, and the biggest thing, he was eating normally. In my opinion, he started getting sicker once that chemo entered his body. I prayed and prayed for my baby to get well.

On Thanksgiving, we stayed at the hospital all day. We were staying with my son no matter what. Shakil was still in ICU with the mask on his face. I didn't like that look, but it wasn't about how he looked, it was about how he felt. It's been five months now, and I didn't see him getting any better. I looked at him, knowing he needed a mask to help him breathe better. I would break down and cry while he was asleep.

CHAPTER TEN

December came, and it was my older son's birthday. I didn't really spend any time with him because I was too busy at the hospital. As I write this now, I never asked him how he felt about that situation.

Shakil's birthday was coming up. I asked him, *"What do you want for your birthday?"*

His responded, *"I want to have a party!"*

"A Party? You are in the hospital. I can't promise you that, but I will see."

The next day I spoke to the social worker about the party. She thought it was a great idea, and I told her that Shakil had come up with it.

Shakil would be turning twelve years old on December 16th. I told him it was okay to have his party. Even though he was still in ICU, we could invite a couple of people, though not too many. I could see he was so excited; everyone was. I asked Shakil, *"What are we going to eat at this party?"* Guess what he said? Hot dogs and chips!

I started thinking about the time when they let him come home for the weekend. When I asked him what he wanted for dinner then, he had said hot dogs. So yes, I had a moment. I asked him, *"Are you sure? Are you going to eat one?"*

He said, *"Yeah!"*

He still didn't have an appetite, so for him to speak about food was surprising. Everyone contributed, even the staff at the hospital. I started calling everyone to let them know about the party. My baby was so excited and I really saw it in his face. I couldn't believe we were planning a party in the ICU! I had so much to do!

Shakil was feeling better, but he still had the mask on. I took it off for one second to hear him talk. He told me to put the mask back on. I wanted to cry; I knew he couldn't breathe without it. I needed something to pick me back up, so I went to put in the order for the cake. I went to the store to get some decorations. I was happy and excited, thinking maybe this was what he needed, family and friends around him.

Two days before his party, he was up playing his game. I was sitting there talking on the phone, making sure everyone would be able to make it Friday. Everything was done; I had everything except the cake. It would be picked up that Friday afternoon.

On Friday, I was cleaning and hanging up the decorations. The nurse went downstairs to have the hot dogs cooked. People started arriving and it was getting too crowded. The nurse said we had to take some of the guests down the hall into the playroom. No more than five people were able to come in the room. They had said to invite a couple of people, and when everyone comes to something you invite them too. I figure you invite twenty people and ten will show up.

We took the food and the leftover decorations to the playroom. Lots of family and friends showed up for the party - more people than I expected. Everyone was having a good time, and even though there was no music, it was still a party.

The cake arrived, and it was time to sing happy birthday. We all gathered around Shakil's bed and sang to him. After that, my husband and I blew out the candles.

Shakil was so happy, although he couldn't really say anything because of the mask on his face. It was time for Shakil to get some rest. I could see that he was tired. We thanked everyone for coming and for the gifts. It turned out to be a nice party, even though it was in the ICU room of the hospital.

Once everyone left, I asked Shakil if he enjoyed himself. Then he removed the mask himself. He nodded his head up and down. My husband cleaned up Shakil's room. I went to clean up the playroom. Visiting hours were over, and now it was time to relax. We took out all of Shakil's presents and started showing them to him. I was kind of worried that he didn't drink anything all day. His foot had been swollen for a couple of weeks, and I noticed that they were still swollen when I started washing him up for bed. He started falling asleep, and I gave him a kiss on his cheek and said happy birthday.

The next day, Shakil woke up and I noticed his feet

were still swollen. I asked him how he was feeling. He said, *"I'm good."*

I was waiting for the doctor to come in for his morning rounds. I wanted to know why Shakil's feet were still swollen. The doctor entered the room and I asked him about his feet. The doctor said the swelling hadn't gone down yet because he's wasn't moving around. He told me to elevate his feet by placing pillows under them.

Within the hour, family and friends started calling to ask how Shakil liked the party. We talked about that a little. Shakil was sleeping off and on all day. I took it as him being tired from the party. While he was asleep, I was watching television and talking on the phone. Everything was going okay that day. Shakil still has no appetite, though, and I was concerned about him not eating again.

CHAPTER ELEVEN

The next day was Sunday. On December 18th, 2005, I was home that morning and the phone rang. This was the day my whole life changed. It was Shakil, calling me - and mind you, he still had his mask on. He wanted to know what time I was coming up there. I told him soon, and I asked him if he was okay.

He said, *"I'm good."*

But one hour later he called me again. I told him I would be up there soon. Another one hour later, he called again. He said, *"Mom, I thought you was on your way?"*

I said, *"I will be up there in a few minutes."* I stopped doing what I was doing and got ready to go to the hospital. My son wanted his mother there, so I was on my way. I was getting dressed when the phone ring again. It was Shakil. I said, *"I'm on my way!"*

He said, *"Come now."* Then he asked me to bring him an iced tea.

Now that was odd. Like I said, he wasn't eating or drinking anything for a couple of weeks. I finally get to the hospital with the iced tea. I gave him a kiss and said,

"You sure you are all right?" He said yes. I asked him, *"Do you want the iced tea now?"* and he said no. I could tell he was happy I was there. He fell asleep and I watched television and talked on the phone.

Shakil woke up around three that afternoon. He lifted his mask up and said, *"Mom, I want my iced tea."*

I poured his tea in a cup and got him a straw. I asked him, *"Does it taste good?"*

"Yeah." A couple minutes later, he had trouble breathing be cause has mask was off. I had to hurry up and put his mask back on.

The next thing I know, around fifteen minutes later, he started vomiting up the iced tea. I had to call for a nurse to come in the room. The nurse cleaned his mask and washed off his face. I kept asking him if he was all right. He wasn't answering me at all. I didn't like his facial expression, so I called my husband and explained to him what had just happened.

I was sitting by his bedside holding his hand. I was so nervous; it was scary. Like ten minutes later, Shakil started vomiting blood. I ran out and called the nurse again. She came in and ran back into the hallway, yelling, *"Someone call the doctor!"*

This time, my heart felt different. He wasn't breathing all that well; something wasn't right this time. I called my husband again and told him he must come to the hospital now. I knew something wasn't right.

A couple of doctors came in and checked Shakil out. My son looked so scared in the face, and I couldn't do anything. I just burst out in tears and asked the doctors,

"*What is going on with my baby?*" He had stopped vomiting, at least, and the nurses were cleaning him off.

My husband arrived at the hospital so fast. I'm sure he ran a couple of red lights. The doctor said to us he needed to take an X-ray of his lungs. I don't know, but it seemed to me he knew what was going on. I was mad at myself because my son needed me and I couldn't do anything. I think I prayed five times within that minute.

The doctor came back with Shakil's results. He asked us to come out in the hallway. I was thinking, "*Here comes the bad news*". You know when the doctor has bad news. You can look at his face and tell. He told us Shakil lungs had collapsed, and that's why he was vomiting the blood. Then he said it didn't look good at all. I just started crying and praying.

Then came the news no parent wants to hear. "*I'm so sorry; your son is not going to make it through the night.*"

I said, "*What you are talking about?*" I heard him talking, but didn't hear him talking. The doctor had repeated himself. I just started screaming, and saying, "*No! No! No! Not my baby! What am I supposed to do without my son? What would be my reason for living? He needs me!*"

We walked back into the room, and I was in a daze. I looked at my baby; he was actually fighting for his life, and on top of that, the doctor just put a time limit on his life. I had to ask myself if there was really a God. If there was a God, why was He putting my child through this? A child should outlive their parents. In today's world, I see a lot of parents outliving their kids.

I showed my son a lot of love. Now it was time to tell him. I sat by his bedside and told him, *"I'm so sorry you are going through this. I love you with all my heart, and you will always be a part of me no matter what."* And I just started crying, saying why. I told him everything would be all right. I felt like I was lying to him because I knew he was leaving my world.

It was getting hard for Shakil to breathe. I had to go in the hallway; I tried not to cry again. I really couldn't hold my tears anymore. *What does a mother do?* I started feeling nauseous and my stomach was hurting so bad. All I could say was, *"Why, why?"*

CHAPTER TWELVE

I looked into the room, and everyone was standing around him. They came back into the hallway, the doctor and my husband. The doctor said to me, *"His heart rate is still dropping."* My husband just shook his head.

As a mother I, didn't want to hear that; it was always bad news. The doctor had the nerve to ask me if he stopped breathing, did I want to put him on a respirator (breathing machine).

I asked him, *"What are you talking about?"* My mind was somewhere else. To answer the doctor's question, I said, *"Yes."*

"Are you sure?"

"Yes," I repeated.

The doctor explained to me what the machine would be doing. He said Shakil would not be breathing on his own; the machine would be doing it for him. All I knew was that I didn't want my baby to leave me. The doctor also said that he would be suffering and eventually he would pass on.

I started thinking, *do I want my son to suffer or do I just let him go?* As a mother, I needed him to be with me. He was too young to die, I mean way too young. I couldn't stand staying in the room watching him trying to breathe. I didn't want to lose him, but he was leaving me, and I couldn't make the cancer go away. I couldn't make him better. He was really leaving me.

I walked back into the room. My husband was sitting next to Shakil, holding his hand. I was crying so hard; I couldn't help it. There was no keeping anything under control. This was reality, and it was killing me mentally. I just kept looking at Shakil's chest to make sure his heart was beating. I had to leave the room again; I couldn't be in there.

The doctor came out in the hallway and said, *"His heart rate is dropping faster than I thought. Do you need to call anyone?"*

I just looked at him. He asked me about the respirator again. I said, *"He doesn't need to be on it."* It hurt me to say that, like I was pulling the plug on him. I remember walking to the nurse's station to call my mom. You know your mother will be the first person you call. I dialed the number and my mom picked up the phone. I couldn't say anything; I was too busy crying. My husband had taken the phone out of my hand and he started talking to my mom. I couldn't tell you what they talked about. My mind was gone; it wasn't there.

I cried and my husband hugged me as we walked back to Shakil's room. My husband stayed in the hallway talking to the doctor. Once I entered the room, I saw

Shakil had trouble breathing. I stuck my head out of the room to call my husband. My husband sat on the edge of his bed. He didn't have that long. I asked myself how a human being can tell a mother that her son can go any minute. No, I didn't at that time think he was just doing his job! I was upset at the doctors, nurses, and really, even God. I really felt at the time that God had let me down. I prayed a lot, more than I ever prayed in my life.

I just kept thinking, *"Does Shakil know he is dying?"* I walked over to his bed and gave him a hug and kiss and told him I would always love him.

My husband was talking to him. He told Shakil, *"Everything is in God's hands; don't fight it. And when I go fishing, you will be there."*

Shakil responded, *"Okay, Dad."*

I ran out of the room and sat in the chair in the hallway. My husband came out and said, *"He's gone."*

It wasn't even two minutes later, and my son's last words were, *"Okay, Dad."*

I headed back into the room and kissed him and told him I love him again. I looked at his chest, and there was no heartbeat. He was gone, he was really gone.

My family started arriving, and as they were walking towards Shakil's room, my husband stopped them and told them the news. I was still in the room. They were taking everything off him like the heart monitor and the IV out his arm. My baby was gone, just lying there like he was sleeping. I kept hoping he would wake up, but he didn't. It was hard to face reality when it was right in front of your face.

I look at it now that God called on another young angel. Back then I didn't believe it, and no one could have made me believe it. Two days after his twelfth birthday on December 18th, 2005, God called on Shakil to come home. After all of this, I was hoping that it was still a dream.

Reality set in. We stayed at the hospital until they took Shakil to the morgue. I was back and forth into the room. I couldn't stay in the room knowing my baby wasn't any longer with me. He looked so peaceful lying in the bed. Everyone in the family started leaving the hospital. I was going nowhere until they took Shakil downstairs to the morgue. We had to wait until someone came to the room to wrap his body. It seemed like I couldn't stop crying. My baby was really gone; this man (meaning the doctor) was right.

I heard someone crying inside the room. I walked back into the room, and it was a nurse. She had been taking care of Shakil since he had been in ICU. She said, "*I can't do this, I will not do this*." And then she walked right out the room.

Before they wrapped his body, I gave him a kiss and said goodbye. They took his body out of the room. It felt like I was going to die to.

As I walked into our apartment, I felt strange knowing that Shakil would not see us or this apartment again. I went into his room, rubbed his pillow, just stood there looking around at his things. I walked in my room, still crying. I was getting ready to lie down. I couldn't sleep all night; you wouldn't believe the things I was thinking about. I was thinking about Shakil, I was wondering if he was cold, did he need a blanket and was he scared? I know it sounds a little crazy. I was still his mother and worrying about him still. I kept tossing and turning; I couldn't sleep for nothing.

I got up and went to the bathroom and looked in his room. His bed was empty; I was hoping all of this was a dream. I asked God again, "Why did you take my baby from me?" I wanted to know. Even though my husband told me I should never question God, I did it anyway.

The next morning the phone started ringing. I was still lying in the bed, looking at the walls. I didn't want to talk to anyone; I didn't want to see anyone. I just wanted to stay in bed all day. I finally got up and went into the kitchen. Yes, I was thinking crazy again. I was wondering if the dishes Shakil ate out of gave him cancer. All types of things was running through my mind.

I just kept hearing the phone ring; it was getting on my nerves. It seemed like everyone was calling at one time. My husband said we had to get in touch with the funeral home. I looked at my husband like I looked at the doctors in the hospital who said crazy stuff to me. I didn't want to talk about a funeral home, insurance, anything! My baby's body wasn't even cold for 24 hours yet.

I went back in the bedroom and got back into the bed. Now I didn't have any appetite. I wasn't thinking about how to plan my child's funeral. I was still wishing he was here.

My husband handled everything. He talked to everyone who called the house. He made the funeral arrangements. I was there, but I was in a whole different world. Let's just say my body was there, but my mind wasn't.

I was still in the bed when I heard my husband talking on the phone, talking about Shakil. I just started crying and closed my door. I couldn't even hear him talk about Shakil. It was too soon for everything. He was just a child; it was too soon. He wouldn't be graduating from high school. He wouldn't be getting married. He wouldn't be having kids. It was just too soon.

CHAPTER THIRTEEN

I felt so drained. I kept asking myself, *"What am I'm going to do without Shakil?"* Shakil was the only person on my mind since he passed away. I just wanted everyone to stop calling the house. It had been a couple of days and nothing changed. I still hadn't eaten anything.

I missed the little things about him. Every morning he would come in my room and give me a kiss and tell me he loved me. He would call me from my mom's apartment to see what I was doing, and before he hung up the phone, he would say, *"I love you, Mom."* It was just the little things, like his smile. Today I will close my eyes just to picture his smile. I'm looking at his picture while I'm writing this book. It's giving me so much strength to complete it.

Give your kids hugs, kisses, and say to them every day that you love them. Don't take life for granted. Tomorrow is not promised to anyone.

We were looking through the insurance policies. That's another thing - life insurance is a must-have. Was I prepared to use the policy? No! But thank God I had life insurance. You have to have life insurance in today's world. It's so much easier to have and a lot cheaper than you think. All we had to do is take it to the funeral home and what they didn't use, they gave it back. It made everything so easy, instead of worrying about how we were going to pay for the funeral.

I was walking around the kitchen again, asking myself, *"How did my son get cancer?"* I started thinking about what the doctor had told me. He had said, *"Remember, Shakil did not die from cancer. He died from an infection he caught. Sometimes the illness doesn't kill you, but the complications do."*

I'd been in the house all week and it was time to get out. We went shopping for the funeral. Shakil was buried in the suit he wore when I got married. It wasn't the same shopping without him. I was hoping I didn't run into anyone. I used to hate for people to say, *"Sorry about your loss."* Every time I heard that it made me cry.

That night I finally turned on the television. I wasn't watching it; I was just thinking. My phone was still ringing off the hook. I finally spoke to my mom, just to let her know I was all right. We had two days until the funeral. Do you know that was hard? The funeral was two days before Christmas. That really sucks to lose someone, but to lose them around the holidays? I really felt like my heart was ripped out my body. If you haven't lost a child, you will never understand how I felt. I had to deal with losing a child and make sure my other child was all right.

I notice I hadn't prayed since Shakil had passed away. I was upset, yes at God! He took my baby away after all the praying I did. He still took him from me. So I asked myself, why continue praying? I realized I needed to do it for us, meaning his family and for Shakil's soul. No matter what, I still had to pray. To this day, I pray every day, especially thanking God for waking me up every morning. I had to learn that life didn't stop because of a death.

The day of Shakil's funeral, I woke up nauseous and nervous. The phone was ringing that morning. The family had started calling to see how we were holding up. I don't think we said one word to each other, and if we did, I couldn't tell you what they were. We were walking out the door and the neighbors were outside talking to my husband. I kept walking; I didn't want to talk.

We got in the limo and drove off. We arrived at the church. I was really scared to get out of the limo. I hesitated at first because there were a lot of people in front of the church. I took a deep breath and got out of the limo. We started walking towards the church, hugging everyone. Everyone kept telling us how sorry they were. I was trying to hold my tears in.

As I sat down, the casket was closed. I just kept looking at it, hoping it was not true. I couldn't really tell you who was there. My mind was focused on my son. A couple of people talked and the preacher did his preaching. The funeral was soon over.

Going to the burial ground, my husband did a good job. He had it set up for the driver to go past our building and the park. They used to fish there all the time. My husband got out of the car and threw some flowers in the water. Then he got back in the car and we pulled off. Finally we were on our way to the burial ground, this time for real. It was a sad day for us. I will never forget that day as long as I live.

AFTER THE STORM

I was a mother who had just lost her son and didn't know what to do. I went through a lot. I started losing a lot of weight and having nerve problems. I didn't want to go back to work. I stayed in the house, and I didn't want to go out. I went to see my doctor and she told me I had to go back to work. She told me I needed to get out of the house. She also said I needed to start eating again, reminding me that I had another son that was alive and needed me.

She was right. I was thinking about Shakil. I still couldn't believe he was gone. Now I was thinking about him lying in the dirt, wondering if ants or any types of bugs could get into his casket. I know it was just a thought.

A week later, I started having throbbing in my head. I didn't know at the time what it was. I had to go back to the doctor. Now I was scared, because that never happened to me before.

The doctor said, *"You are back?"*

I started smiling. I explained to her what was going on with me.

She examined me and said, *"It's your nerves. You have to let it go. I know you love your son, but this is not healthy. You are going to kill yourself. Start thinking, about happy things."*

I asked her, *"How? I miss him so much! All I do is think about him when I wake up and before I go to sleep."*

She said, *"I know you have to get better."*

But, in reality, she didn't know. She had never lost a child before, so how would she know how I felt? That was impossible.

She said, *"I don't want to put you on any medicine because it could be addicting."*

I hate taking medicine anyway; I didn't want to be put on anything. She advised me to go and talk to someone or go to a support group. She gave me a list of names and numbers to check out. No! I didn't call or go see anyone. I tried to handle it on my own. I can say this, though: you do need to talk to someone that has been through what you are going through as far as losing a child. If that person you are talking to didn't ever lose a child, it's not going to work, because they really don't understand your pain. Go get help or join a support group. I know, I'm telling you to do this when I didn't. Just trust me. The real reason I didn't see anyone is because, just like I said, if they didn't lose a child, they would not understand my pain. Plus, I'm shy. I don't like talking in front of a crowd.

One thing my doctor was right about was going back

to work. I went back to work and it did help. I was so busy at work that I really didn't have time to think. My job really kept me busy.

At home, I was still having nerve problems. This time I felt the jumping in my arms and leg. I would be scared to go to sleep, afraid I wasn't going to wake up. A week later, I went back to the doctor again and she said the same thing, that it was nerves.

She said, "I don't really want to give you medicine, I really don't. You really have to relax. This is getting serious now. You really, really, need to relax. I don't want to see you in my office again anytime soon. The next time I will prescribe you something to relax you."

I still had the same problem for at least a month. All I did was just pray and ask God to give me strength to get through this. Guess what? He did. In reality, if it wasn't for God giving me that strength. There was no way in the world I would have written my first book "*What Does A Mother Do? The Shakil Williams Story!*" And now be on my second book. Even though a big piece of my heart was taken from me, I'm blessed. Things happen for a reason, and I'm learning that today. You can't control the impossible; all you can do is hand it over to God.

A couple of weeks later, we received a call from the County Executive of Newark, NJ telling us that they were having a ceremony in May in honor of my son. Going back to the day of the funeral, the County Executive did speak at my son funeral. He said he was planning on naming the kids' playground after my son in Branch Brook Park in Newark, NJ. I never thought twice about it.

A lot of people were saying a lot of things. Getting back to the phone call...the secretary was giving us all the information about the ceremony. I was surprised that he kept his word!

The day of the ceremony, it was packed in the park. The set-up was great. They had chairs and flowers everywhere. Everyone was walking up to us, shaking our hands. I was so happy about the ceremony. Our families started showing up. I was happy to see a familiar faces. We sat down to listen to everyone speak, and it lasted about one hour. At the end of the show, we went over to the opening of the kids' playground. We looked up and it said Shakil Williams Playground. I just started crying and hugging my husband. That was really an honor to our family.

It wasn't over yet. We stepped over just a little to the right and he had an American flag covering something. He pulled off the flag and it was an engraved rock. It was like we were dreaming. That was a big turnout. Until this day, the Shakil Williams Playground is still standing tall. If you are ever in Newark, NJ, go past and see the dedication.

A week later, I put a thank you card in the mail. Ever since then, we've been giving a big event in the park, giving back to the kids. I know Shakil is looking down on us, so proud of us.

It took me a long time to give some of his things away. I didn't get rid of anything until it was time for me to move. I was going through his things; I wanted to keep a lot of them. I know it was time to give them to someone. I was crying going through his clothes, remembering the day he had this on, the day he had that on,, when I bought him this. It was hard going through his things. Nothing was harder than burying him. A mother shouldn't have to bury their child. I still have a couple of his things; I just can't get rid of them. They mean a lot to me. I didn't have a younger child to give his things to.

It's going on eight years. Everyone was right - time does heal, but time took a long time for me. Everyone heals in their own way. I'm still feeling some type of way. I had to re-live it twice. This is my second time writing about him. I'm okay now. I will always have the memories; they are not going anywhere.

By the time a couple of months had passed after the ceremony, my nerves started calming down. We decided to go to the burial ground. I was also nervous about that, but I was more scared than nervous. Everything turned out fine. We prayed and talk to him. I was wondering if he knew we were there. I think his spirit was there with us. We try and visit his grave when we can.

Shakil Williams, 1993-2005... It was a blessing for me to have had Shakil in my life for twelve years. In those twelve years, I can say he lived his life to the fullest. He did a lot of things that other kids couldn't do. I'm proud to say Shakil is my son. He will be missed.

What am I doing eight years later? Well, I moved into my house. I wrote my first book, titled *"What Do A Mother Do? The Shakil Williams Story!"* Every year we give an annual event in Branch Brook Park, in Newark,

NJ to give back to the kids. I have my own blog talk radio show. I'm working on my non-profit organization to help families with children who are battling childhood cancer. Hopefully when this book comes out, I will already have my organization.

I'm just keeping out the negative people and bringing in the positive people.

I will keep on writing; I have a lot on my mind.

We all go through our ups and downs, our sadness and happiness, our good days and bad days, but we always keep it moving. When you lose someone close to you, like a child, it changes everything. It changes the way you look at life. It changes how you live your life. You just look at the world and everything around you differently. I never in a million years believed that things happen for a reason. Now, I do believe it!

To all that are going through a child fighting cancer or have a child that has passed away from childhood cancer, you are not alone. I know you feel alone but you are not. You have to take it one day at a time. I know what you are saying - trust me, I was there. Time does heal, and if you don't believe it now, you will later. Trust me.

Thanks for reading my story, sharing my pain, allowing me to empower you and watch me become an advocate for childhood cancer awareness, not only for my son Shakil, but for all children in the world.

DEDICATION FOR SHAKIL WILLIAMS

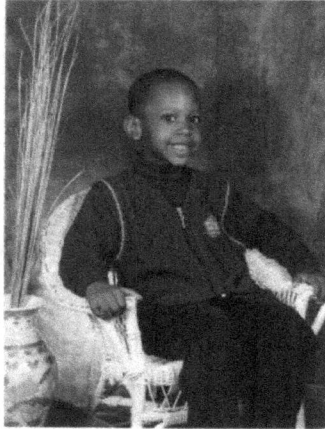

My son, Shakil, was everything you would have wanted in a child. I'm so sad that cancer had to be a part of my family life. I dedicate this story to him. I know he's looking down on me and proud that I'm sharing our story. Shakil loved fishing. He won the kids' Fishing Derby eleven times within a couple of years. He loved wrestling, and he never missed a show. He loved playing the video games, like PlayStation. He had so many game cartridges. One other thing he loved doing was going outside to play with his friends.

I knew what he really loved doing the most, and that was spending time with his family. Shakil was so funny; he was always clowning around. He was always making people laugh. I just knew he was going to grow up and be a comedian.

Shakil was a true trooper. Shakil is and was a winner. He did not lose his battle to cancer. He won. He won because he never lost sight of what was important: his family and friends. Shakil never gave up. He was a fighter to the end. Shakil will always have a place in my heart and he will always be missed.

I love you, Shakil!

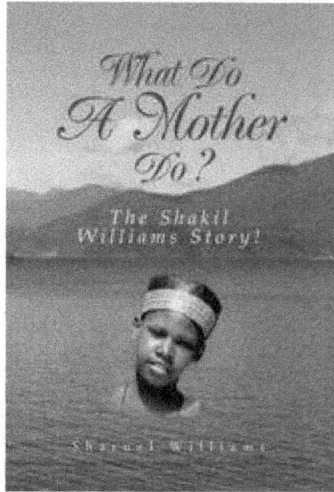

BIO FOR SHARNEL WILLIAMS

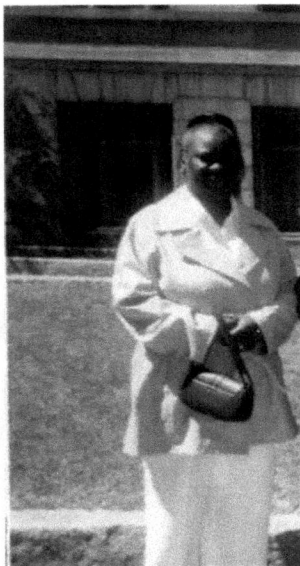

My name is Sharnel Williams. I was born and raised in Newark, NJ. I'm a wife, mother, grandmother and author. I'm the oldest out of seven kids - two girls and five boys. I started writing my first back in 2006, a couple of months after the passing of my son. My first book is about my son battling cancer. This will be my second book published and my first anthology. I'm also working on my third book. Currently, I'm working on starting my own non-profit organization to help families with a child who has childhood cancer. Here are ways to contact me:

- www.facebook.com/sharnelw
- www.whatdoamotherdo.com
- www.twitter.com/authorsharnel
- www.blogtalkradio/authorsharnel

NYASIA'S STORY

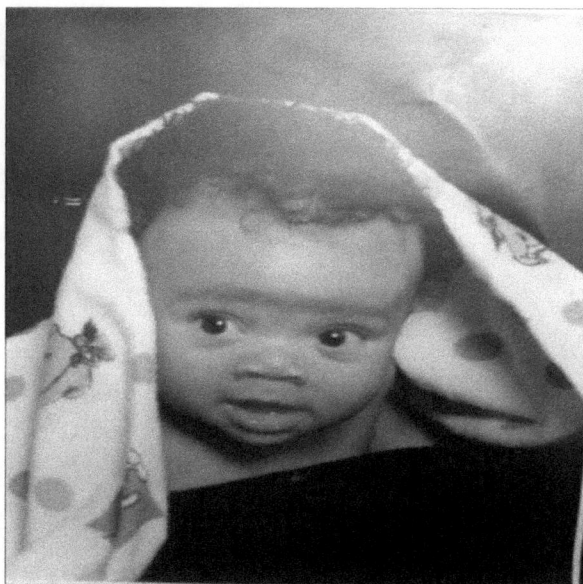

A True Story By:
Nicole Martin

ACKNOWLEDGEMENTS

It was only by the grace of God that this story was written. I would first like to say thank you to Sharnel Williams for coming up with this beautiful idea and including me on this project. I have grown so close to you and Carla that it feels like we have known each other forever. You guys are truly a great team to work with and I love y'all so much. There were so many times I felt like giving up and throwing in the towel writing this, but having y'all to talk too made me push harder to get through this project.

To my sister Sabrina, you were there with me and loved my Nyasia as much as I did. I thank you for being a part of her/my life.

To my family and friends that loved her and never treated her differently, I thank you.

To everyone that had a part in caring for Nyasia, her teachers, school bus drivers, aides, doctors, nurses; I thank you so much for always handling my baby with so much love.

To Mr. Rodney Wilkins…sometimes we don't know why the things that happen in our lives happen, but I know we should never question God. I love you so much, and the way you took to my daughter from the moment she met you was nothing but pure love. You taught me that it was okay to travel with her, even by bus, train, etc. You did it with no problem and never once complained. You came into our lives and immediately became her father, the only father she ever knew, and for that, I will always love you.

I wrote this story to give other parents a glimpse into my life and to hopefully help someone else cope with similar circumstances. My contact information will be listed on my author page. This book is for whoever is reading it, and I thank you in advance for taking time out of your life to spend a day in mine. To all my readers, I thank you for reading my story.

CHAPTER ONE
INTRODUCTION

Can you imagine having to raise a beautiful baby girl and having her suddenly taken away from you without warning?

Well, that's what happened to me. I had no idea my baby was about to leave me. I would give anything to hold her in my arms one more time or to get one of the big, juicy kisses she frequently would give me. I have to give all thanks to God for allowing me to care for such a beautiful child, for allowing her to grow inside me and become a part of me for twelve years.

Here is my story...

"Lord, please don't let this doctor tell me that what I already know." Those were the last thoughts I remember having before having my pregnancy confirmed. *"What's next? How in the world could I let this happen?"* I was not ready to have another child. I was already struggling with the one that I had. This couldn't have come at a worse time in my life. It hurts to tell this story as raw and

truthful as I am about to tell it, but not only will I let you into my life, but my ultimate goal is to free myself of all the pain and frustration I have held inside me for so long. I pray that none of you will ever have to experience all the pain I did with losing a child that I not only carried inside me for nine months, but also loved unconditionally. Without warning, I woke up one day and found my baby dead in her bed. *Can you imagine*? I hope and pray you never ever have to experience that kind of hurt. Here is my story – and Nyasia's…

CHAPTER TWO

I can still remember the day I went into labor. I was staying with my mother temporarily because the apartment I'd lived in was infested with field mice - one critter that I don't play games with and refuse to live with. I still wonder how long those things were in my apartment because it wasn't until I was nine months pregnant that I got wind that I had them. My stepfather, Mr. John, was nice enough to go to my apartment to set traps, seal holes, and promise that he would get rid of them after failed attempts with the maintenance department of South woods in Essex. He and my mom suggested that Daneira (*my three year old*) and I come stay with them temporarily until the problem was fixed.

That particular day, Saturday, November 1, 1997, I needed to run home to get some things from the apartment. Mom really didn't like the idea of me driving alone since I was due to deliver any day, but I felt that I would be okay, so I went on my instincts. When I got there, I'd checked my phone messages, mail, etc. and grabbed a few belongings. I was on the phone chatting with my friend when I felt a strong need to use the bathroom. Once I sat to pee, I felt a huge gush of fluid escape me and I immediately knew that it was my water breaking.

When I stood, the fluid kept dripping and I was unable to control it. However, I didn't feel any pain at all so I figured I would have time to get back to my mom's to drop my bags off and go to the hospital. Once I'd packed everything that I had come to get, which took less than ten minutes or so, I placed a bunch of tissue and a maxi pad into my underwear, jumped in the car, and headed to Cedonia where my mother resided. I did call her to let her know what was going on.

My mother was very afraid to drive the Beltway, and since that was the quickest route to my house, she seldom came to Essex. She was very afraid that I would out of nowhere begin contracting and she wanted me to pull over and call an ambulance. I refused and I made it to her house. We switched cars and drove to John Hopkins. My Aunt Leona was there and she stayed back with my daughter Daneira.

Once I was admitted, it took no time for my cousin and her best friend to come and be a part of the birth of my baby. Even though I wanted to smack both of them for coming into my hospital room with my favorite food from my favorite sub shop, "*Mama Mia's*", and the aroma of a freshly-made cheesesteak was making my stomach flip. I was still happy that they were there.

On top of teasing me with food, both of them grabbed

recliners and turned to face the small color television which was currently airing some episodes of *Martin,* and the two of them couldn't stop laughing. You had to love them though. They were there, and that was all that mattered. As I cried out in agony, they remained laughing and eating away at their food as if I wasn't there. I couldn't do anything but smile inside because it was funny when I thought about it.

CHAPTER THREE

"Pushhhhhhhhhhhhhh!"

That was the last thing I remember hearing the doctor say before giving birth to a healthy baby girl. Nyasia Alexis Martin came into this world weighing 9 lbs. 3 ounces with a nose that spread across her whole face. The doctor put her into my arms and I remember thinking "Eww!" because she wasn't the cutest infant I had seen. But it didn't take long before I fell deeply in love with my baby. I'd learned that Nyasia had split me from front to back so I had to get a whole heap of stitches.

As soon as I got into a deep sleep, I was awakened by the nurse bringing Nyasia to me to feed, since I'd requested no formula. I knew exactly what to do, since it wasn't my first time breastfeeding. I did notice my baby had a much stronger grip on me then I'd remember Daneira having.

Just as I finished feeding her, we got an unexpected visitor, the one person that I didn't expect to see in a million years - Nyasia's father. When he walked in, I was just laying her back into the glass bassinet provided by the hospital. I felt how strong his eyes were on me, but I refused to look up at him. He had made it very clear that he wasn't interested in having a baby with me when I got pregnant with her. He and I had started dating in my senior year of high school and were kind of on and off. Neither of us was really ready to be in a committed relationship, and if he told the story, I am sure he would tell it differently. He frequently told me that it was my fault that we didn't work out because I was still in love with my oldest daughter's father. In all honestly, he would be right.

When he took one look at Nyasia, he made mention of how light she was. *"She is light as a light bulb, it's no way she is my baby. She is too light."*

I wasn't in the mood to argue with him. He didn't take into consideration that I was light and I came from a light, damn near white family. He picked Nyasia up out of her bassinet and held her for a few before handing me a gift bag filled with all sorts of baby stuff for her. After staring at her for what seemed to be forever, he left and told me he would be back the next day. However, that day never came.

The next morning, I was awakened to a team of doctors coming into my room and telling me that they had some concerns about my baby. Their exact words were that something wasn't quite normal with her and that they wanted to run some tests on her. I cannot remember if I'd asked them about the tests or not because I was so out of it from the meds I'd constantly received intravenously. I do remember awakening later and asking where my baby was and the nurse telling me that the doctors had her and that she would be back to me shortly. When the doctors bought Nyasia back, they assured me that everything was fine and that they would inform me of any findings as soon as the test results came back.

I spent the rest of that day with my family and friends that visited us. It was wonderful having so many people come and shower us with their presence and gifts for both of us. I knew that I was loved and that I had a bond that couldn't be broken because my family and close friends always had my back. Nyasia was set and there wasn't anything that I needed for her. Later that evening, I was told by the doctors that Nyasia had a touch of newborn pneumonia and possibly meningitis and that she would have to stay in the hospital awhile. However, I would be discharged in the morning.

"There is no way in the world I am leaving this hospital without my baby!"

The doctor couldn't believe my reaction. I can't remember every single thing I said to her, but I can say it wasn't good because they had to get security to try and calm me down.

The last person I remember laying eyes on was my mother. They were slick to call her because she was the only person that was able to talk some sense into me, reminding me that I had a three-year-old at home who needed me too. I finally gave in and was discharged the next morning, but I didn't leave the hospital. I went straight over to the nursery and stayed there until visiting hours were over. I think this was the point when the hospitals began to allow overnight visits to parents. I cried so badly that the doctors made a room for me to be able to stay there with her.

The next morning, a different team of doctors came in to let me know that Nyasia was being discharged on a program called "*Home Health Care*" and that it was important for me to allow the nurses and doctors to come and treat her for the remainder of her treatment plan.

CHAPTER FOUR

As months went on, I began to realize that Nyasia wasn't meeting her milestones. She wasn't doing the things that I thought a baby her age should be doing and she was very colicky. I bought my concerns to her pediatrician, who in turn told me that all babies grow at their own pace and that I would need to have more patience with her.

As Nyasia grew older, it became evident that she was different. Her doctor finally recommended a program called "Infants and Toddlers" to help with her physical and social developments. She wasn't meeting the milestones that she should have, and by time she turned two, she still wasn't walking, talking, or making eye contact with me or her sister. Her social skills were nonexistent and all she wanted to do was eat, sleep, and watch Barney.

I felt like I'd become a prisoner in my own home because she hated to be out in public places. She would act out in ways that weren't considered normal for a baby let alone a child period. I'd seen children falling out and acting up in stores and stuff, but this was different.

I was an investigator. The doctors would tell me that she would grow out of it, but I knew in my heart that it was something definitely wrong. I did a lot of research on the internet and tried remedies such as reducing sugar intake and taking her off dairy products, but none of these things seemed to work. Then I came across something on the internet that taught me about autism. I was sure that was what my baby had and I immediately contacted her doctor to tell her about what I'd learned. The doctor took into consideration what I'd said and set Nyasia up for testing at a place called Kennedy Krieger Institute, which was a hospital geared towards meeting the needs of children with disabilities.

The time had come for Nyasia to go to her appointment. It was super scary seeing all the doctors come in the room looking at her and asking me the same questions over and over again. They would examine her and write notes on their pads. One would leave, and a few seconds later, another would come in and do the exact same thing. After hours of collecting information and testing/examining her, I was finally led to a room with Nyasia that looked more like an office setting then a hospital room. I was told to have a seat, and there was a lady sitting next to me with a doctor sitting behind a desk where a computer was held.

The doctor informed me that my daughter had been diagnosed with severe mental retardation or in other words, she was severely developmentally delayed. I was told there was a chance that she would never walk or talk and that she would need to use a wheelchair. *"She will always be dependent on care and will never be able to live alone."*

I felt like my world had come to an end. No! This couldn't be happening. I thought I was coming here to get her fixed! Why were they telling me these lies! I wasn't about to believe anything they were saying! *"Doctor, is there anything you can do? Anything? I can raise money!"*

The doctor just shook his head no as the lady tried to console me.

"There are places that are equipped to handle a child like yours and you would be able to see her anytime you want."

That statement echoed in my head over and over again. I did not realize the severity of what it was that they were really saying.

"No! She is my child and she isn't going ANYWHERE!" I grabbed Nyasia and walked out of the clinic, telling the valet to get my car quickly so that I could take my baby far away from there. First they sprang news like that on me, then they gestured to take her. No! I absolutely hated those people and didn't want to be in their presence any longer then I had too.

Once I had gotten in the car, I called my mother to let her know what the doctors had said. She asked if I needed her to meet me somewhere. I didn't want to be around anyone but my baby. I was still in shock. I had no idea what life had in store for me and I was scared. I looked back at Nyasia, who was looking out the window smiling and waving her hands in the air. I tried to digest everything I had learned, but I just couldn't. I couldn't understand why it was happening. I didn't smoke, drink, or do drugs. I went to all my prenatal appointments. I just couldn't understand why something like this was happening to me. As time went on, I was able to accept the fact that my baby wouldn't be able to perform all the normal functions that another child her age would. Nyasia was a delight to have. Even though at times it was difficult to care for her, I loved her with all my heart, and I was finally able to accept the fact that she wasn't perfect. If anyone had to describe her in one word, most the time the word "love" came to mind. She never attempted to bring harm to anyone. She always smiled and showed love to her family and she was actually a joy to be around. She did love her own space, though. She didn't like to be crowded and she wasn't comfortable around strangers or in strange places. I think she sensed that people were afraid of her, especially kids whom didn't know how to take her.

We had moved into a small townhome which was still larger than the apartment we were living in and closer to Daneira's school. The kids around the community weren't that friendly with Ny, but it was okay. I didn't expect everyone to welcome her with open arms. As long as they didn't bring danger or harm to my child, then the comments bothered me less and less.

It did start to have an effect on her sister though. She would frequently become angry and didn't want me to stroll her around the neighborhood because of the comments children would make. It took a while before Daneira was able to accept that her sister was different and that we had no control over what others thought about her. She was ours, and I wasn't about to make her a prisoner in her own home because of some disadvantaged children who weren't taught respect.

CHAPTER FIVE

Nyasia formed a bond with her sister that would forever remain. As time went on, Nyasia began to crawl and she eventually began to walk. She was starting to do all the things that doctors said she wouldn't do. This gave me a huge glimpse of hope. Nyasia even started to say "da da". Thinking back to how I felt when I heard her say that, knowing that she didn't have a daddy around, added another stress to my heart because I felt like my baby deserved to have someone to call Daddy. I remember reaching out to her father to no avail.

My mother would tell me to let that dream go. *"Nyasia is a gift to you from God. He would only give his special angels to those he knew would love and take care of them, and he chose you."*

My mother was right. I remembered hearing time and time again that God wouldn't place anything on us that we couldn't handle. However, I was becoming lonely and depressed. I felt like something in my life was missing because I wasn't happy. I can remember going to bed crying at night, wishing that I had someone to help me and give me time to enjoy my own life. It was the same boring routine every single day. Back in the late 90's, there weren't many people onto having home computers, but I can remember making it one of my best friends. See, there was no Myspace, Facebook, or social networks where you had friends/family members that were accessible to talk to right away. Furthermore, most of my family and friends were working, so I was left to be home alone with my daughter a lot. My routine was to get up and get Daneira ready for school, and then I would spend most of the day with Nyasia. I wasn't able to hold onto a job because all the babysitters I would get for Nyasia would frequently quit on me, which made me in turn unable to work. I can still remember the one time I thought I had found the perfect daycare provider for her. She told me that she had experience with children with special needs, and I took Ny over to meet her and she seemed so loving and friendly. I was starting a job assignment with a temp agency and I was excited. I would finally be able to do normal things and make money and stop living off of Section 8 and government assistance.

However, after a few days of Nyasia being dropped off to her, she quit on me. The funny part was that she didn't give me a warning or anything. I guess I tried to ignore and brush off the sighs and stuff she would do when I would pick her up. One morning after dropping Neira off, I arrived to her house and she wouldn't answer her door for me. I knew she was there because her window was open and I'd just heard her chatting on the telephone. She even went so far as to whisper to someone to be quiet and take the other kids downstairs.

As I went to put Nyasia back into her car seat, I could feel the lump forming in my throat and the anxiety building up inside as I tried my best not to cry. When I got to the driver's seat, I could no longer hold it in. I cried frantically like a baby right there in front of her door. As I write this story, I can remember this cold wind coming across me and it was like I heard God talking to me.

"Stop crying! I will make a way out of no way! Don't you worry, my love, I will always have your back!"

As time went on, there was still something I couldn't quite put my finger on. If I had to give a summary of what I was concerned about, I would say that Nyasia seemed to fiend for milk! It was like she would actually shake when she saw me pouring it, and when I would go to hand it to her, she would gulp it down so fast that it almost seemed unhealthy. When I bought this to her pediatrician, she thought I was overreacting and basically brushed it off, saying that she was born a big baby and she probably just had a huge appetite. She didn't seem to take into consideration that I wasn't saying she was like that with all things (food, juice, snacks, fruit, etc.), it was only when she saw milk.

Being the investigator that I am, I searched the internet for answers, and I was amazed at some of the things that I saw some parents saying about milk. There were lots of people expressing the same concerns as me, saying there was an addictive ingredient in milk. I read stories where parents would actually completely remove milk from their child's diet and saw remarkable results!

It was another glimpse of hope - or so I thought. I decided to remove the milk from Nyasia's diet. After a couple of months, it was evident that I was getting the same results and that Nyasia basically just craved more juice. I began to feel like I was getting nowhere, but the answers were out there. I felt like I was in a world of my own, stuck, and left to find the answers without any help.

I remember having a conversation with my sister about everything. She was the one person I could depend on to take Nyasia and give me a break every once in a while, however, she worked crazy hours as a Correctional Officer and she had a child herself who had some medical issues, so it wasn't that often that she able to get her. She eventually moved directly across the street from me, and Lord knows she made my life a whole lot easier at this point. I no longer had to worry about taking Nyasia places she wasn't comfortable with, for example, Supermarkets, Wal-Mart, or Shopping Malls. And since my sister worked second shift (*3pm until 11pm*), she didn't mind watching her and letting me run errands during the day before she would go to work.

CHAPTER SIX

"Mommy! Mommy! Quick, come here! It's Nyasia!"
I still remember the frantic call for me as I was sleeping a little later than normal on a summer morning. Daneira sound so nervous and scared and I didn't know what to expect as I jumped out of my bed and headed to her and Ny's room. Nyasia was laying in her crib shaking and trembling. Her tongue was hanging down the side of her mouth and she didn't appear to be conscious. I quickly screamed for Neira to grab the phone and dial 911.

"Operator, my three-year-old daughter is shaking and trembling and I believe she is having a seizure!"
The operator asked a few questions and I began to get upset, thinking that she needed to be sending someone instead of questioning me about my child. I wasn't aware that she already had someone on the way to me and was just keeping me on the phone and helping me help my daughter until they arrived.

We were taken to Franklin Square Hospital in Baltimore County, where Nyasia was examined and transferred to John Hopkins. She was diagnosed with having a seizure, however, the doctors couldn't tell me whether or not it would continue. I was basically told if she had anymore, then I could bring her back. Otherwise, I would need to make an appointment with her pediatrician right away.

At that point, I decided it was time to look for a new doctor for her, because in my opinion, her doctor wasn't knowledgeable enough to give medical care to my daughter. I think this was the best decision yet I'd made, because my investigative ways made me interview doctors and ask about their experience with children like Nyasia before I made a choice.

I carefully chose a doctor that I felt could handle her needs: Dr. Theresa Pugh from John Hopkins White Marsh. She took to Nyasia right away. She was very caring and Nyasia even seemed happy around her. Dr. Pugh sent Nyasia back to Kennedy for additional testing and she also gave me a referral for her to see a neurologist. She even sent her for testing on her heart, eyes, and genetics. She didn't want to miss anything, and she listened to all my concerns and didn't brush any of them off. She wrote notes as we talked and shared her experiences with other children like Nyasia. I felt like I'd finally found the one. She would email me over time and ask about Ny and would have her staff check on her from time to time to make sure that Nyasia and I both were okay.

After completing the test rounds at Kennedy and being giving the same diagnosis she was given back when she was one, Nyasia went to see her neurologist. His name was Dr. Eric Kossoff in the John Hopkins Outpatient Center and he brought in a team of doctors including the top surgeon, Dr. Weingard, as they accessed my baby. She was sent for an EKG and other testing. I was told that Nyasia had some abnormal activity going on in the left side of her brain which might cause her to have seizures. She was also given a diagnosis of macrocephaly. After looking the term up, I saw that it meant that she basically had a large head. Her doctors suggested surgery where they could place a tube in my baby's head which would drain off excess fluid from her brain, since she was borderline to have a condition called hydrocephalus.

I listened to them talk to one another, and in my opinion, they didn't all seem to be on the same page about the surgery. I was told that they would contact me on the decision and a tentative date for surgery. Now let me kind of go back a little in this story to give some background. I have a nephew who was about a year and a half older than Nyasia that was born with a condition called hydrocephalus.

Through my research, here is what I learned:

Hydrocephalus is an accumulation of fluid within the cranium, especially in infancy, due to obstruction of the movement of cerebrospinal fluid, often causing great enlargement of the head; water on the brain.

Macro cephalous is being or having a head with a large cranial capacity and/or being or having a skull with

97

a large cranial capacity.

I shared that with you because I want you to be able to see the similarities in the diagnosis of both me and my sister's children. I figured okay, maybe it's in the bloodline and maybe I should go along with what the doctors suggest.

However, I wasn't totally convinced that Nyasia needed surgery. My nephew Anthony was diagnosed with the condition at birth and had to have the surgery before he turned one. With all my research, hydrocephalus is usually diagnosed right away and my daughter's wasn't. I just felt in my spirit that I should get another opinion, so before I'd given the doctors an opportunity to call with a surgery date, I emailed my concerns to Dr. Pugh, who in turn scheduled Nyasia for a second opinion with one of the top neurologists in the world. She did warn me that it would take a while for her to be seen because Dr. Ben Carson was one who people traveled from across the world to get seen by.

When Nyasia's appointment date came around, I can remember feeling so much anxiety. I was so nervous and scared. I mean, it was something I had thought about on a daily basis during the seven months I waited for this day to come. Can you imagine having to keep so many feelings bottled up inside you, not having a mate to talk to or hold you and let you know that everything would be okay?

I'd also started working during this time. I had landed a job with a wonderful non-profit agency called Families Involved Together. Their goal was to advocate for parents and caregivers of children with special needs, and a job requirement was that you had to either have a child with special needs or care for one. It was only by the grace of God that I came across the posting for this job. It was perfect for me, and I'd claimed it before I even went for my interview. Nyasia had started going to school and she was picked up Monday through Friday at 10:50 a.m. by a school bus. She didn't return home until about 5 p.m., attending a Baltimore County school by the name Ridge Ruxton.

My job allowed me to work around her schedule and even do some hours at home. It was PERFECT! Daneira was going to Elmwood Elementary full time and I'd even found a daycare provider that lived a few doors up from me who was able to keep both of them until I got off work on the days I would stay late. She, too, had a child with a disability, and although she didn't know much about Nyasia's diagnosis, she was willing to learn how to care for her. I remember her telling me that Daneira pretty much did everything for Ny and taught her how to care for her pretty well too. Besides, I would never work any later than 5 p.m. unless it was a support group or workshop that I was facilitating.

Everyone that was close to me was so anxious to hear what Dr. Carson's recommendation would be for Nyasia. I remember wondering if he would be able to do something to make Nyasia be able to talk and do things that I saw other children her age without disabilities doing. *Maybe he could give her some sort of medicine or something,* I thought.

Dr. Carson was very friendly and upbeat and had a way of making us feel super comfortable. Daneira was about six or seven years old and she went along with me to the appointment.

Dr. Carson had all of Nyasia's records, her cat scans, MRI's, and EKG results. He sat next to me and played with Ny a little and smiled at her and then at me. He shook his head no. "Your daughter does not need surgery. She does have a slightly elevated size in head for her age, however, as she grows, it will not be noticeable at all. She just has a big head! Look at you, your head isn't that small either!"

I burst into laughter at how wonderful he made me feel at that moment and he even added the humor to his report. As he continued speaking to me, asking if large heads ran in my family, he pulled out a measuring tape and measured Nyasia's, Daneira's, and my head. We all fell into a category of having a head size larger than our ages. Dr. Carson did tell me that there was a possibility that Nyasia would develop frequent seizures due to the amount of activity going on in her brain "However, we would deal with that if and when the time comes."

When I asked if there was anything he could do to prevent it, he told me that if there was, he would be scheduling a procedure or prescribing medication right now. However, due to the extreme activity and the places where it was happening, it would be too dangerous to do surgery. He recommended that I keep being the concerned, loving parent that he was sure that I was and that if anything changed to contact his office for another

appointment. He also wanted Nyasia to continue seeing Dr. Kossoff every six months. I was happy! I felt like me paying attention and speaking my concerns paid off. I didn't want my baby to have to go through a brain surgery. I remembered how I felt when I was by my sister's side when she went through it, and it was emotionally draining. As time went on, I became accustomed to my routine and I felt better about life. I was working and making good money. I was in a program with Department of Housing where they would allow a certain amount of the income paid towards rent to be placed in an escrow account over a course of five years and they would give it to you at the end towards the purchase of a home. Nyasia was comfortable in her daycare setting and Daneira was happy as well. She was making new friends in our neighborhood and frequently invited to different events throughout the community.

Although Fontana wasn't the best place to live, it was comfortable and there were people like us in the neighborhood. My neighbors and I looked out for one another, especially when it came to our children. Now there were the ones that would make it uncomfortable for me to take Nyasia out to play. They lived in different courts in the neighborhood and would come around and make fun of her. I will never forget the day my daughter's school bus pulled up to drop her off and a load of kids bombed the bus with snowballs, laughing and making fun of all the special needs kids on the bus. My heart melted as I became enraged, wishing for a moment that God would allow me to go back in time to become their age so that I could beat the mess out of every last one of them.

Daneira would chase after them in anger and scream and call them names, and I had to remain the adult and try to calm her, all the while going through the emotions I felt internally. I secretly hated them and sometimes wished bad things would happen to them. I am being totally honest about my feelings, I know it wasn't right for me to feel that way but I am sure any parent can relate being in my shoes at that moment. I wondered what type of parents raised them because they were so cruel. It had gotten to the point that the bus driver would have to have police escort them into the community to drop my daughter off. I felt embarrassed and sometimes afraid that they would try to come in my home and harm my daughter. However, I would never let it show. I did make a few calls to some family members their ages to come scare them off.

I continued with my life and continued bottling these feelings inside me. I remember I started to become extremely close with my family, particularly my cousins, and they knew that it was hard for me to get out to outings so they would frequently visit me and stay around to keep me company on the weekends. Sabrina was only off like one weekend out of a month so I couldn't ask her to always use it to watch Nyasia.

My cousins added excitement to my life. They would come over and we would play cards, charades, and karaoke and have all sorts of fun. Even though I had two children, I was still a kid at heart and I enjoyed our times of acting silly and having fun.

My family gave a family reunion every year that still goes on to this day during the Labor Day holiday and I looked forward to getting away and spending time with them. Even though things seemed to be looking up, I still felt like there was something missing in my life. I did go out on dates, but I yearned for the attention of a man to call my own secretly while telling others I didn't have time for a man in my life.

I never thought the day would come that I would find a soul mate, but little did I know that it would sooner than I thought. I had just arrived at work and my supervisor didn't let me get good and seated at my desk before handing me an intake form, telling me to call the parent. He gave me all the details about him, saying that he had a son that had an eye disorder and cerebral palsy and that he was interested in getting some resources for him. Robert (my supervisor) also told me to make it a priority.

I got right on the call. I noticed on the form that it was a father, which wasn't common. Most of the parents that called in for assistance were women. There was something about the phone call that was different than any other call I had taken. The parent agreed to come to a workshop we were holding at the center a few days away, and from the moment I laid eyes on him, I felt like love at first sight truly existed.

After the workshop, as I went to issue him his certificate of attendance, he asked if I could write down my personal number so that he could take me out sometime. I went against all company rules and did it, and we are still together to this day.

When he met my daughters, he took to them right away as they did to him. He never once treated Nyasia any differently and became very keen to learn about her and her medical issues. He would take Nyasia to playgrounds and swing her on the swings, which she loved to do. If other kids would say something negative about my daughter, he had a way to look at them and make them go about their business. It wasn't long after we met that we moved in together, and shortly after, with our combined income and the money I'd earned from the housing program I was in that I mentioned earlier, we moved to a better community that wasn't far from where we were. My children were able to stay in there same schools. My financial situation was getting better and better, however, the worst was yet to come.

CHAPTER SEVEN

As time went on, Nyasia began to have more seizures, just as the doctor warned me. It had gotten to the point where she had to use a wheelchair to travel and even a helmet for protection to avoid head injuries. On top of that, I was given notice by my job that I would soon be laid off because the funding for our program had been cut. Years had passed and I was no longer receiving any type of government assistance. My rent was over a thousand dollars a month and I had just recently purchased a SUV, so I had a payment of over three hundred dollars along with car insurance. I had no idea what I was going to do; I was scared. My boyfriend was in a program and wasn't able to support me financially at the time, so once again, I started to feel scared, nervous, an anxious.

For a while, I was able to turn to family members to help keep us from being evicted and winding up homeless. But that was short-lived, of course, because who could really turn to family to help every single month? I was receiving unemployment, but it wasn't enough to pay the bills, and since my boyfriend was no longer working, his income had stopped as well. I lost my SUV first and shortly thereafter I lost my home and had to move back in with my mother with my children. I was so depressed and I had found a way to mask my feelings by secretly indulging in alcohol and drugs, unbeknownst to my family.

Months went by and I'd finally gotten another job. I'd lied on my application, saying that I had a bachelor's degree in special education, and I was hired to be a "Special Needs Counselor". I lasted there for a whole year and kept my secret to myself. The only other person that knew for certain was my fiancé Rodney. Many would say that if I hadn't met him then I would have never taken that route, but I beg to differ. When I look back on my life and all the risks I would take, such as selling weed in high school and preparing fraudulent tax returns just so that I could feed my children and myself and to stay above water, even getting caught and doing time. None of that stopped my behavior. I was a risk taker and I was known to do the things I wanted to do. I felt like the cards I had been dealt in life were so unfair that I didn't care about the consequences of any of my actions – or so I thought. However, I wasn't prepared for the day that my children would be taken from me.

When I knew in my heart that my habit was getting the best of me and I needed help, I cried out for it. I asked for the help of my sister and my mother while I got myself together, but all the back and forth led them to go get legal custody of my children. Sometimes I wonder if my decisions affected Nyasia's health, because the times that I would see her, it seemed as if her condition worsened even more.

She was finally documented as having epilepsy and placed on medication. I was so back in forth in her life that I decided it was time for me to give myself a long stretch of time and get it together so that I could go back to caring for my children. They were heartbroken. Daneira would express her feelings verbally to me but Nyasia's hurt was all in her eyes and in her body language. However, she would still light up when she would see me.

Daneira's father was a part of her life and he'd even taken her to live with him in NC for a period of time. This definitely placed a huge strain on my heart, but I knew that I had to get myself healthy for me. Otherwise, it wouldn't work.

After spending a year in a program, I was finally able to regain stability for both myself and my fiancé. We were both working again and we moved out of the recovery homes we'd lived in and back into a home where I was able to regain custody of my children. Nyasia had actually been living in a group home for children with special needs out in Silver Spring, MD.

My sister had gotten to the point where she could no longer handle caring for her. I remember getting the phone call while I was at Warwick Manor that my daughter was being placed in foster care. I cried like a baby and I hated and resented my sister for sending her there. I hated knowing that she had to be cared for by strangers, and I felt none of this would have never happened had I not made the bad decisions I had made. I was there for all the right reasons. However, this was an extra boost for me to do what I had too to get my daughter back in my care.

CHAPTER EIGHT

After signing my new lease to a three bedroom home, I decided that although I was super anxious to bring Nyasia back home, I wanted to have help in place. I couldn't allow myself to fall back into the stressful pattern of living and wind up back in the situation I was in. I reached out to so many agencies and finally I got a call back from this program out in Woodlawn called PACT. They had what was called a family support service for families of children with severe disabilities.

I was assigned a case manager, Mr. Winn. He was a Godsend because he addressed every single one of my needs in that one visit and promised me that as long as I did my part with recovery, he would do his part in making sure that I wouldn't have to take this journey alone. Mr. Winn meant every single word of what he said. I was given an allowance of forty hours of care per week, one weekend a month of respite care, and family allowances toward things like rent, gas, electric, and food.

Nyasia came home within one week of me moving into my new home. Daneira moved in the same day I did. She couldn't wait to get back under my roof. Even though she was extremely close to her grandmother, who she was now residing with, she wanted to be home with her mommy, and since we moved directly across the alley from my mother, she had the best of both worlds and she was happy.

I would be lying if I said I didn't make any mistakes from the time Nyasia moved back in with me up until the time she passed away, because I did. I made many. However, I put my children first and from that day forward, I vowed that they would never leave my care again. I would never put anything before them and I kept my word.

Nyasia's seizures had gotten so bad from the time she left my care throughout my sister caring for her and her living in the group home that she had to be placed on a special diet called a "Ketogenic Diet" to help control them. She was now wearing a protective helmet twenty-four hours a day, and instead of her having just one specific type seizures, she was now having several. I had a lot of research to do, and with me working part time, I had little to no time to myself.

Nyasia had loss so much weight, and in my opinion, she looked unhealthy. I didn't like what I was seeing, so I scheduled an emergency visit with her doctor shortly after she moved back in with me. I wanted to know if the diet she was on was making a difference in her seizure activity and because I'd read about the Atkins Diet also

110

being close to the Ketogenic Diet. The Atkins Diet would allow her to eat a little more. I asked about switching her. Her neurologist was a little skeptical, however, he told me it was my choice.

I immediately took her off the Keto and placed her on Atkins. Since neither the group home nor my sister kept a record of her seizure activity, I had to go off of their guesses. I used a composition notebook to keep track of the seizures that I witnessed and I hired two in-home aides since I was now able too.

I'd noticed within a few weeks that her seizure activity dropped and she was down to less seizures than she was before coming into my care. In my opinion and the opinion of a few others close to me, I think Nyasia was happy to be back with me. She was going back to her school and surrounded by the people who loved her unconditionally. To me, this, along with her medication and diet, was all a part of her treatment plan, and it worked.

She did have her moments when she would have bad days and had to use this medicine called "Diazepam" when she would have five or more seizures within a one hour. It wasn't often at all that she had to take it, and I hated giving it to her because she would be so out of it. It was a powerful drug, a benzoin, and it would make her extremely lethargic. As time went on, the milligrams would increase because her system would become immune to the dosage. I remember asking her neurologist at one of her appointments if there was anything else I could give her that would do the same job but have less of that type of effect on my baby. I then found out that there was. It was called "Ativan", and it too would make her drowsy, however, he prescribed her the lowest dosage possible and told me I could switch it up when need be.

Nyasia would have several more EKG's, and the results showed that there was so much activity going on that it would be almost impossible to completely stop her seizures. It had gotten to the point that I could almost predict when the seizures would come.

I went through so many in-home care providers. It was super hard to find someone who was experienced with handling the many types of seizures my daughter would have. I felt like my sister, Rodney, and I were the only three that knew what to do and how to take care of my baby. Nyasia would have the grand mals that would make her fully unconscious and the drop seizures where out of nowhere, her whole body would forcefully drop. In my opinion, that was more dangerous than the grand mal because if she wasn't wearing a helmet, it would do serious damage to her, especially her head with the way she would drop. Then there was the staring, where it would look as if she was daydreaming. These would happen mostly in the morning when she would be awake. She would drool a lot when they happened and look as if she was staring into space. When she would come out of them, she would let out a huge sigh and began to make her signature babbling sounds. I know this all sounds like a lot, but honestly, Nyasia wasn't really a hard child to care for. The only thing she yearned for was food, love, and affection, and more often than the typical child, she yearned for Barney. My baby had every Barney episode you could name. She even sometimes had double episodes because I wasn't the only one purchasing them for her. She had my mother, my sister, and even sometimes her teachers purchasing the new Barney movies because they knew how strong her love was for that character. It was weird though that anytime Barney came to town and I would take her to the shows, it wouldn't keep her attention!

CHAPTER NINE

It seemed as if time was flying by the way Nyasia was growing into a beautiful young lady. She developed a tight bond with her sister and with her cousin Anthony. Even though she couldn't speak verbally, she had her ways of telling everyone what she wanted and we all understood.

Financially, things had once again become tough for me and forced me to have to leave the home I lived in across from my mother. We actually wound up moving to a housing project out in Brooklyn Homes. The neighborhood was rough however, the actual house we lived in was beautiful. It was a refurbished home with new everything. We even had a wheelchair ramp for Ny and everything was on one level.

It was so spacious, bright, and clean! When we first moved there, I absolutely loved the home and so did Ny. She loved her new bedroom and the space she had to move around. The one thing I didn't like about the home was that it wasn't carpeted. I was very concerned about that and tried numerous times to get carpet installed. I felt it was a dangerous because of the type seizures Nyasia had.

I did wind up having to transfer her to city schools, which was something else I hated to do. However, it turned out not to be so bad. Mr. Winn was by our side through the whole adjustment process. He even rented a U-Haul for us to move our stuff.

Rodney lived with us for a while but he eventually moved to Woodlawn to live with his own children. Daneira was totally against the idea of living in the projects, so she begged to stay back with my mother so that she could stay at her school and be close to her friends. Who was I to make her come? In a way, I felt like I was a prisoner in my home because I wasn't able to do much. Ny didn't like being out in public places. I had to work around her school and therapy schedules, so it felt wrong for me to make her come. I allowed Daneira to stay with my mother.

The entire time I lived in Brooklyn, I found ways to numb my feelings. I hated that I'd gotten to the point that I had to live in the projects and I knew in my heart that this wasn't the plan God had for me. Even though Rodney didn't live there with me, he made it his business to check on me every single day. He came over and made sure that we were okay and stayed overnight often.

One morning I awoke to my normal routine of taking Ny to the kitchen after brushing her teeth, washing her, and dressing her for breakfast. She was wearing her protective helmet and walking to the kitchen as I normally would let her do. As soon as she turned to go into the kitchen, my worst fear came to light. Nyasia had a drop seizure that basically forced her body to the hard-paneled floor and she began to shake vigorously. I secured her to make sure nothing sharp was near her and to let the seizure take its course.

As she came out of the seizure, I noticed blood coming from her head and swelling above her eye. I immediately called 911 and she was rushed to Harbor Hospital. Harbor realized the impact was too great for them to care for and they called John Hopkins to pick up their patient.

JHH rushed in and got us care in a blink of an eye. Nyasia had suffered a concussion and had to have surgery because she was bleeding internally. She spent a total of five days in the hospital before she was discharged home with me, and she was given even more round-the-clock care.

During this time, I learned about a bed that Nyasia was eligible for that would keep her from falling while she was asleep and she was even given a better wheelchair. I started to feel like, "*Why did it take bad things to happen before she was given the care and tools needed to care for her?*" The bed was called a "Posey Bed". I recommend this bed to any mother/caregiver out there that has a child who suffers from seizures. There had been so many times Ny would fall out of her bed while sleeping from having seizures that there were too many to account for. I couldn't believe none of health care providers had told me about it. The only way I learned about it was because during her stay at Johns Hopkins, they'd realized just how hard it was to keep her safe, so they ordered the bed for her while she was there and I'd asked if there were a way I could get one for her at home.

Nyasia's recovery process from the incident was slow, but she tolerated it well with the help of the medication and having me there for her around the clock. I have to add that it was very overwhelming. The extra care from the providers really sucked because so many times, they would call off or not show up when they were supposed to. I would have to rely on family members, particularly my sister and Rodney, to help out more than the providers did. One particular nurse aide, "Ms. Rosalyn Fontah", was a Godsend. She even began to go to school with Nyasia every day, so she was her personal nurse to make sure that my baby was safe at all times.

CHAPTER TEN

The kids in Brooklyn Home were just as heartless as the ones I mentioned earlier in the story. They began to do things that were totally unacceptable to treat a person the way they did. They threw things at my baby as she got on and off the school bus, and they threw things like watermelons at our front door. They even went as far as opening her screen in her bedroom and throwing water balloons inside. How could children be so cruel, and who was raising these monsters? This went on for some time during my short stay at Brooklyn Homes. I had to get my baby away from that horrible place.

Sad to say, I only lasted there for a little under a year before I decided it was time for me to move. Although I wasn't at my best financially or emotionally, I was determined to find better living arrangements for us. Rodney was now working full time and he welcomed the idea of me moving away from that area, because he was totally against it from the beginning. He even offered to sign a lease for me in a better area. I knew Essex was affordable and it was closer to my family, and I knew the schools were a whole lot better because I'd lived in the area before. We wasted no time packing up and moving to a two bedroom apartment in Hartland Village.

Although my apartment was a lot smaller than the bungalow I lived in out in Brooklyn, I felt a lot safer and better about myself. Daneira continued to live with my mother and stepfather up until we endured a family tragedy.

My mother was diagnosed with breast and lung cancer when Ny was about four years old. She had been living with it for a total of about six years before God called her home. My mother passed away September 23, 2009. We were informed by her doctor that she didn't have long and she was taken to a hospice place where she lived for two days before passing.

Daneira immediately packed up and moved in with me. I was now driving at this time, so she was able to stay in her same school. She was now a sophomore in high school. My responsibilities had gotten to be greater than I was able to handle, and once again I'd gotten scared and began to mask my feelings. Looking back, I would say these were the worst moments of my life because I felt like God had placed way more on me than I was able to bear. I wasn't working anywhere, and I was now responsible for the care of both my children. I had no job but had rent and a car payment. I had a way of digging myself in holes so deep that it would be almost impossible for me to pull out of.

But through it all, my faith was so great, and although

I didn't know how I was going to do it, I knew it was going to be done. My mother had left behind a policy that was enough for me to pay my rent for a few months and get ahead in my bills until I could figure a way to do what I needed to do to make sure that we were okay. Rodney too was a blessing. He was living straight (drug and alcohol free), working full time, and he had my back despite the many mistakes I would make.

CHAPTER ELEVEN

It had been eight months since my mother had passed and I'd manage to keep afloat in my apartment. My sister lived within walking distance from me and she often called for me to bring Ny over to her house. This particular evening, I wasn't feeling up to it, and I felt physically and emotionally drained when she called for Ny.

Although I would have love to have a little break, I was being lazy, and on top of that, something just told me to keep Ny home with me.

Daneira was visiting with her father in NC for a few weeks, then she was going straight to New Jersey to spend a few weeks with her aunt and her cousins.

Daneira was now five months pregnant as well. When I found out she was pregnant, I knew I had to stay on the path because I was about to become a grandmother on top of everything else I was dealing with. Thinking back to the day Neira left, I'd notice she kept going back to her room and kissing Ny repeatedly saying goodbye to her. It was almost like she knew that it would be the last time she would see her alive.

Thursday, June 24, 2010 at approximately 8 a.m., I got a wakeup call from Rodney. I laid in bed and talked with him for a few before I looked over at the clock, realizing how late it was. I was known as the early bird. I had a routine of getting up about 7 a.m. so that I could be up right before Ny. I had about a half hour to myself before washing her face, brushing her teeth, feeding her, and giving Nyasia her meds. Ny seldom slept past 8 a.m., so I decided to go in and check on her. I was still on the phone talking to Rodney when I went in her room.

"LEMME CALL YOU BACK!" I slammed the phone down, unzipped her Posey bed, and noticed the discoloration in her face. I touched her and felt how cold her feet were.

I immediately called 911 and screamed to the operator that I think my baby was dead. "SHE IS COLD AND HER FACE IS BLUE!"

The operator begged me to keep calm and do as she said while help was on the way. She coached me through CPR and as I did it, I could hear the sirens. I ran to unlock the door, and when the ambo techs ran to her room, I heard total and complete silence. One tech walked out to me and shook his head, and I remember letting out a scream so loud that I knew everyone in my complex heard.

I can't even type all the feelings I felt when I heard them requesting for the coroner to come. The ambo tried to calm me down, but I couldn't stop screaming and crying. I felt like my world had come to an end. I couldn't believe my baby was gone. I heard a female tech saying that she appeared to have vomited and possibly choked. Nyasia was known to vomit after a grand mal seizure. The coroner asked me tons of questions about her and asked what type of health issues she'd had because they saw she was wearing a helmet, they saw her wheelchair, and saw that she was in her Posey bed. When I told them she had a seizure disorder, they shook heads in agreement that she must had had a seizure in her sleep.

After I'd called Rodney - and I hated to tell him that over the phone - I called my sister. I can't quite remember if I told her that it was Ny because I had begun to break down again. But I remember the ambo lady telling her there was a death in the family and if she could, to get around here with me as soon as possible.

From that point, I had no idea how my family found out. All I knew is that they were all there in the blink of an eye. My grandmother, my sister and nephew, Rodney, my stepfather and my aunts, cousins, and my friend Tish and her sister-n-law Robin all came. Robin gathered us all in a circle and said a prayer for me. I don't even think I was able to stand for it. The tears wouldn't stop flowing. I felt like I was having a bad dream and it would all be over soon. I do remember thinking hard about Daneira. I hated to have to tell her over the phone, but because the news was traveling so fast, I couldn't allow my daughter to find out through a social network like Facebook. I could hear the agony and screams through the phone when I told Daneira that her sister passed away. Treina,

Daneira's Aunt, agreed to bring her home right away.

After the coroner cleared her death from any type suspicion, I was asked if I wanted her transported to a particular funeral home. I remember my grandmother answering for me: *"Take her straight to March's Funeral Home"*.

I knew my mother had life insurance for Ny, but since I hadn't been paying on the policy, I wasn't sure if it still existed. But to my surprise, it did. I was able to give my baby a beautiful home-going service. Please if you don't have insurance for yourself and your children, get it. It's very important and it lessened the financial burden of funeral/burial cost. Nyasia was buried right next to my mother too. When I look back on everything today, I am thankful that she no longer has to endure the horrible seizures.

Rodney spoke about her at the funeral, and one thing he said that stuck was that Nyasia was formed out of nothing but pure love. She never uttered a bad word about anyone and loved everyone. There was no better way to describe who she was, he summed it up in that short phrase.

AFTER THE STORM

Today as I write this story, it has been three years since my baby left this earth. I know that she is all around me. Not a day goes by that I don't think of her. I have been blessed with two beautiful grandbabies, Janiyah and Autumn. They are a constant reminder of her because I look into their eyes sometimes and see my baby. I guess it's true that God doesn't make any mistakes. I always say that Nyasia is in heaven smiling down on me with my mother and father.

While I never had a chance to actually hear my daughter talk, she came to me in a dream shortly after her passing to say goodbye. It felt so, so real! I could see her so clearly and she told me that she wanted to say goodbye but she didn't have a lot of time. The kisses I gave her felt so real. Sometimes I go to sleep praying to God that she comes to me again. While I have had dreams about her since that visit, none of them felt the way that one dream felt.

I know my baby is proud of me. I am now a successful

published author of four books, two of which are anthologies (this one included), and I am finally stable. I have her pictures posted all over my home and she is with my parents.

I do look forward to seeing my baby again. They say some have to go for others to live, so I guess that was the case because Janiyah came into my life shortly after Ny's passing and I latched on to her as if she was my own daughter instead of granddaughter. If you or someone close to you is experiencing the loss of a child, I am here to tell you that the healing process isn't an easy one. But time really does heal all wounds. There will always been a place reserved in my heart for my daughter. I wish so many times that I could hear her signature sound, or be greeted with one of her big hugs and kisses, however, I know we will meet again.

Rodney and I are still together to this day, planning for our wedding, and we are both in recovery and doing very well. I no longer live in the apartment. I now live in a townhome and my sister is still not far from me. Each year on November 2nd (Nyasia's birthday), we go to her gravesite and share memories of her and let go of balloons for her. It's a very special occasion, because not only do we get to visit her site, we get to visit my mother's because she is right next to her. ☺ One thing I want to add is that Nyasia was called home June 24, 2010, while my father was called home June 24, 1995. How ironic is that? To me it goes to show that God makes no mistakes.

The End...

DEDICATION TO NYASIA

Nyasia Alexus Martin

Sunrise: November 2, 1997   Sunset: June 24, 2010

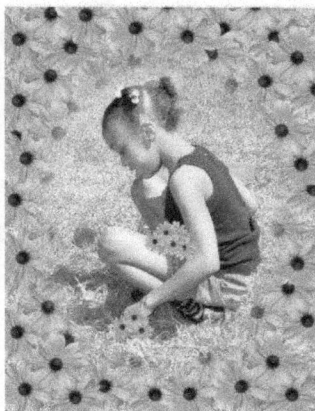

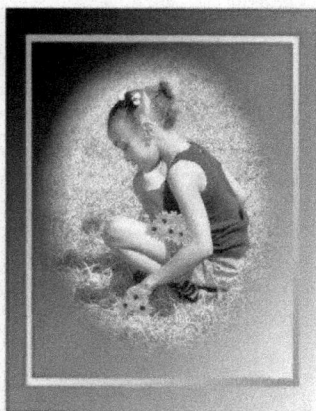

Not a day goes by that I don't think of you.

I love you so much and you will forever hold a place in my heart. You spread your wings and flew away.

I know you're in a better place and that place you will stay. Mommy will always think of you until the day we meet again, my love. I will always hold you close in my heart. I thank God for giving me a chance to raise such a beautiful child.

Love Always,
Mommy

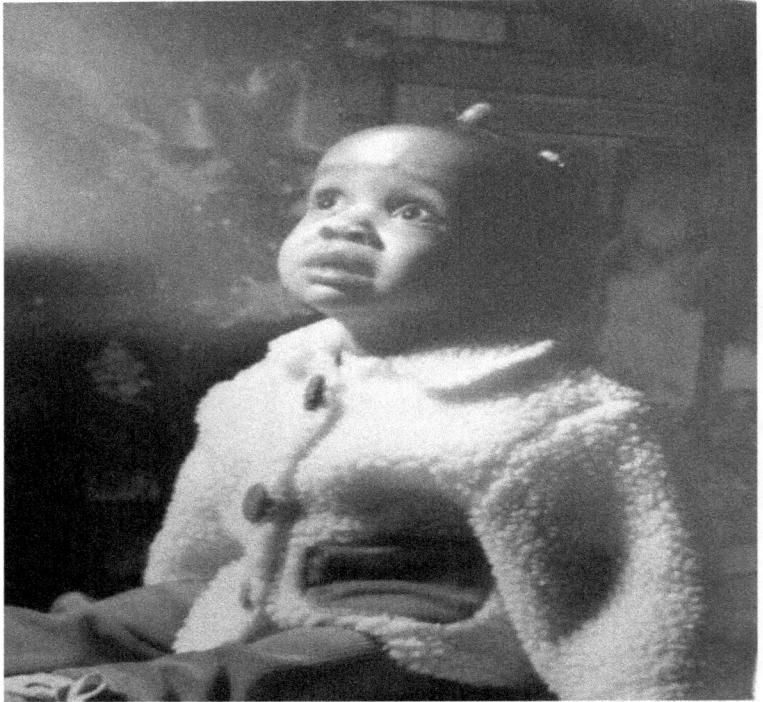

BIO FOR NICOLE MARTIN

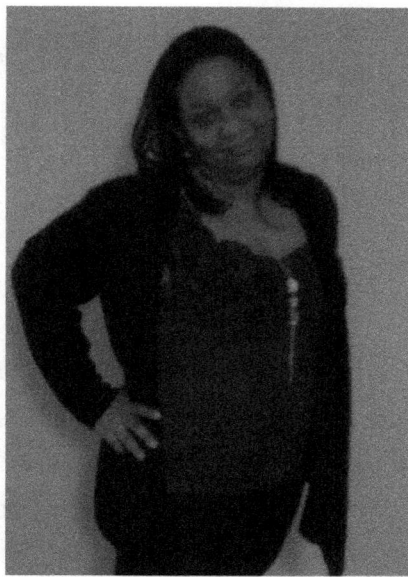

Nicole Martin lives in Baltimore, Maryland with her family. She has two self-published novels entitled "Loving an Addict" and "Poison". She is also featured in an anthology, "Almighty Dolla", where her story was picked up by a publishing company and released. You can buy her books on Amazon, Barnes and Noble, Smash words and Books a Million to name a few.

Here are ways you can contact Author Nicole Martin:

- www.facebook.com/nicolejmartin307
- Instagram – A_NikkiNicole
- Twitter- A_NikkiNicole
- www.pngpublishing.net
- Crystile22@gmail.com

FROM THE AUTHORS:

We would like to thank you for reading our stories. It wasn't easy for either of us to re-live these moments. We pray that our goal of helping someone has been reached. Losing a child is never easy, however, God saw fit to call our angels home. While we know that God doesn't make any mistakes, it doesn't stop us from missing them.

If you know someone whom our stories can benefit, please share our title with them. We put this together in hopes of helping others and we want our story to reach people all across the world. Check out our trailer on YouTube by typing in "A Mother's Worst Nightmare...Read Our Stories, Share Our Angels."

Again, we thank you for your support and for taking the time to read our stories.

Sincerely,
Nicole and Sharnel

www.ingramcontent.com/pod-product-compliance
Lightning Source LLC
Chambersburg PA
CBHW051043030426
42339CB00006B/168